Medical Heretics and the Fallacy of the Expert

How the medical establishment crushes the truth and suppresses good ideas

Vernon Coleman

Vernon Coleman: What the papers say:

'Vernon Coleman writes brilliant books.' – *The Good Book Guide*
'No thinking person can ignore him.' – *The Ecologist*
'The calmest voice of reason.' – *The Observer*
'A godsend.' – *Daily Telegraph*
'Superstar.' – *Independent on Sunday*
'Brilliant!' – *The People*
'Compulsive reading.' – *The Guardian*
'His message is important.' – *The Economist*
'He's the Lone Ranger, Robin Hood and the Equalizer rolled into one.' – *Glasgow Evening Times*
'The man is a national treasure.' – *What Doctors Don't Tell You*
'His advice is optimistic and enthusiastic.' – *British Medical Journal*
'Revered guru of medicine.' – *Nursing Times*
'Gentle, kind and caring' – *Western Daily Press*
'His trademark is that he doesn't mince words. Far funnier than the usual tone of soupy piety you get from his colleagues.' – *The Guardian*
'Dr Coleman is one of our most enlightened, trenchant and sensitive dispensers of medical advice.' – *The Observer*
'I would much rather spend an evening in his company than be trapped for five minutes in a radio commentary box with Mr Geoffrey Boycott.' – Peter Tinniswood, *Punch*
'Hard hitting...inimitably forthright.' – *Hull Daily Mail*
'Refreshingly forthright.' – *Liverpool Daily Post*
'Outspoken and alert.' – *Sunday Express*
'Dr Coleman made me think again.' – *BBC World Service*
'Marvellously succinct, refreshingly sensible.' – *The Spectator*
'Probably one of the most brilliant men alive today.' – *Irish Times*
'King of the media docs.' – *The Independent*
'Britain's leading medical author.' – *The Star*
'Britain's leading health care campaigner.' – *The Sun*
'Perhaps the best known health writer for the general public in the world today.' – *The Therapist*
'The patient's champion.' – *Birmingham Post*

'A persuasive writer whose arguments, based on research and experience, are sound.' – *Nursing Standard*

'The doctor who dares to speak his mind.' – *Oxford Mail*

'He writes lucidly and wittily.' – *Good Housekeeping*

Books by Vernon Coleman include:

Medical
The Medicine Men
Paper Doctors
Everything You Want To Know About Ageing
The Home Pharmacy
Aspirin or Ambulance
Face Values
Stress and Your Stomach
A Guide to Child Health
Guilt
The Good Medicine Guide
An A to Z of Women's Problems
Bodypower
Bodysense
Taking Care of Your Skin
Life without Tranquillisers
High Blood Pressure
Diabetes
Arthritis
Eczema and Dermatitis
The Story of Medicine
Natural Pain Control
Mindpower
Addicts and Addictions
Dr Vernon Coleman's Guide to Alternative Medicine
Stress Management Techniques
Overcoming Stress
The Health Scandal
The 20 Minute Health Check
Sex for Everyone
Mind over Body
Eat Green Lose Weight
Why Doctors Do More Harm Than Good
The Drugs Myth

Complete Guide to Sex
How to Conquer Backache
How to Conquer Pain
Betrayal of Trust
Know Your Drugs
Food for Thought
The Traditional Home Doctor
Relief from IBS
The Parent's Handbook
Men in Bras, Panties and Dresses
Power over Cancer
How to Conquer Arthritis
How to Stop Your Doctor Killing You
Superbody
Stomach Problems – Relief at Last
How to Overcome Guilt
How to Live Longer
Coleman's Laws
Millions of Alzheimer Patients Have Been Misdiagnosed
Climbing Trees at 112
Is Your Health Written in the Stars?
The Kick-Ass A–Z for over 60s
Briefs Encounter
The Benzos Story
Dementia Myth
Waiting

Psychology/Sociology
Stress Control
How to Overcome Toxic Stress
Know Yourself (1988)
Stress and Relaxation
People Watching
Spiritpower
Toxic Stress
I Hope Your Penis Shrivels Up
Oral Sex: Bad Taste and Hard To Swallow
Other People's Problems

The 100 Sexiest, Craziest, Most Outrageous Agony Column
Questions (and Answers) Of All Time
How to Relax and Overcome Stress
Too Sexy To Print
Psychiatry
Are You Living With a Psychopath?

Politics and General
England Our England
Rogue Nation
Confronting the Global Bully
Saving England
Why Everything Is Going To Get Worse Before It Gets Better
The Truth They Won't Tell You...About The EU
Living In a Fascist Country
How to Protect & Preserve Your Freedom, Identity & Privacy
Oil Apocalypse
Gordon is a Moron
The OFPIS File
What Happens Next?
Bloodless Revolution
2020
Stuffed
The Shocking History of the EU
Coming Apocalypse
Covid-19: The Greatest Hoax in History
Old Man in a Chair
Endgame
Proof that Masks do more Harm than Good
Covid-19: The Fraud Continues
Covid-19: Exposing the Lies

Diaries and Autobiography
Diary of a Disgruntled Man
Just another Bloody Year
Bugger off and Leave Me Alone
Return of the Disgruntled Man
Life on the Edge

The Game's Afoot
Tickety Tonk
Memories 1

Animals
Why Animal Experiments Must Stop
Fighting For Animals
Alice and Other Friends
Animal Rights – Human Wrongs
Animal Experiments – Simple Truths

General Non Fiction
How to Publish Your Own Book
How to Make Money While Watching TV
Strange but True
Daily Inspirations
Why Is Public Hair Curly
People Push Bottles Up Peaceniks
Secrets of Paris
Moneypower
101 Things I Have Learned
100 Greatest Englishmen and Englishwomen
Cheese Rolling, Shin Kicking and Ugly Tattoos
One Thing after Another

Novels (General)
Mrs Caldicot's Cabbage War
Mrs Caldicot's Knickerbocker Glory
Mrs Caldicot's Oyster Parade
Mrs Caldicot's Turkish Delight
Deadline
Second Chance
Tunnel
Mr Henry Mulligan
The Truth Kills
Revolt
My Secret Years with Elvis
Balancing the Books

Doctor in Paris
Stories with a Twist in the Tale (short stories)
Dr Bullock's Annals

The Young Country Doctor Series
Bilbury Chronicles
Bilbury Grange
Bilbury Revels
Bilbury Country
Bilbury Village
Bilbury Pie (short stories)
Bilbury Pudding (short stories)
Bilbury Tonic
Bilbury Relish
Bilbury Mixture
Bilbury Delights
Bilbury Joys
Bilbury Tales
Bilbury Days
Bilbury Memories

Novels (Sport)
Thomas Winsden's Cricketing Almanack
Diary of a Cricket Lover
The Village Cricket Tour
The Man Who Inherited a Golf Course
Around the Wicket
Too Many Clubs and Not Enough Balls

Cat books
Alice's Diary
Alice's Adventures
We Love Cats
Cats Own Annual
The Secret Lives of Cats
Cat Basket
The Cataholics' Handbook
Cat Fables

Cat Tales
Catoons from Catland

As Edward Vernon
Practice Makes Perfect
Practise What You Preach
Getting Into Practice
Aphrodisiacs – An Owner's Manual
The Complete Guide to Life

Written with Donna Antoinette Coleman
How to Conquer Health Problems between Ages 50 & 120
Health Secrets Doctors Share With Their Families
Animal Miscellany
England's Glory
Wisdom of Animals

Dedication
To Antoinette: the kindest and gentlest of God's creation; beautiful in body, mind and spirit and loved forever.

Contents

Part One
Experts with Feet of Clay

Members of the establishment always believe they know best and that their experience, their knowledge and their position give them the right to make decisions and to rule. That is why they are known as the establishment. The *Oxford Dictionary of English* definition of 'the establishment' is 'a group in society exercising power and influence over matters of policy, opinion, or taste and seen as resisting change'. It is those words 'resisting change' which are the most significant. Anyone who questions the establishment must, by definition be ignored, and if they persist and seem likely to become a nuisance they must be crushed, suppressed, vilified and ostracised.

The praetorian guard for the establishment consists of 'the experts'.

We are constantly being encouraged to put our faith in experts. The world is controlled by them. They appear on television, on the radio and in newspapers and magazines. Most of them follow the official line on whatever their speciality is supposed to be. They do court appearances for huge fees, acting for the prosecution or the defence. They are quoted in advertisements and many will promote anything if the fee is high enough. A good number rarely practice, teach or write about their subject once they become professional experts. Blessed with government approval they don't think they are right, they know they are right and they behave accordingly. Lobby groups and public relations bodies keep lists of suitable 'experts' who can be relied upon to stick to the officially approved line on almost any subject. Drug industry lobby groups, for example, will provide journalists with 'rent-a-quote' experts who will support the industry point of view on almost anything and provide a quote or an interview at a moment's notice.

But there is plenty of evidence to show that experts (particularly those who are employed, accepted and promoted by the establishment) aren't always terribly reliable. Indeed, a little research shows that they are predictably and reliably unreliable in all areas of endeavour. They tend to hide behind jargon which they use to disguise their ignorance and to convince non-experts that they know more than they do.

In the first part of this book I'm going to show how and why we should retain a modicum of scepticism when experts tell us things – particularly when those experts are part of the establishment. It's vital to remember that so-called experts are often wrong. Indeed, it is no exaggeration to say that they are wrong more often than they are right.

I've collected together a few examples of errors which now appear laughable but which were influential when they were first shared.

So, to start with, in the world of military endeavour the experts can make quite extraordinary misjudgements which may have damaging far-reaching consequences. In 1939, a military expert reassured European politicians that Germany couldn't possibly overcome the Polish cavalry. A month or two later, the Polish cavalry was crushed by the Germans. In 1941, a man called Captain T Pulleston, a former chief of US Naval Intelligence stated that the Hawaiian Islands were 'over-protected'. He predicted that the entire Japanese Fleet and Air Force could not threaten Oahu. The Secretary of the Navy at the time duly reassured the world that whatever happened, the US Navy was not going to be caught napping. And when the officer in charge of radar at Pearl Harbour was informed that the Navy's equipment indicated that at least 50 planes were approaching he replied: 'Well, don't worry about it, it's nothing.' Just before the Japanese attacked Pearl Harbour, the American Government sniffed at worriers and told them they were hysterical to imagine that Japan might contemplate going to war against America.

Financial experts are no better.

In 1929, in America, distinguished financiers queued up to dismiss the chances of there being a stock market crash. And when there was a massive crash they queued up to say that everything was fine again. Bernard Baruch, a distinguished financier, announced that the financial storm had definitely passed. The Harvard Economic Society repeatedly said that a severe economic depression was outside the range of probability. The Society only stopped repeating this nonsense when they ran out of money, because of the depression, and had to stop publication of their journal.

And as the 20th century continued, so financial experts continued to get things badly wrong. In 1959, the managing director of the International Monetary Fund announced that world inflation was over. In 1958, the magazine *Business Week* reassured American car makers that the Japanese car industry wasn't likely to sell many cars in the USA.

Every year, without fail, economic forecasters and highly paid analysts jostle for the chance to show just how ignorant they are, and inept they are at forecasting. And it's widely accepted, even within the financial services industry, that throwing darts at the stock market listings would produce more winners than taking any notice of the plethora of professionals providing investors with advice. I know of professional advisors, widely regarded as experts, who haven't been correct for decades – but who still continue to sell their advice for enthusiastic, amateur investors. Whether their advice is for the short term or the long term, for bonds or for shares, for one country or for the world their only success is in being wrong.

In 1899, the commissioner of the United States Office of Patents urged the President to close down the patent office on the grounds that everything that can be invented has been invented. In 1901, Wilbur Wright told his bother Orville that man wouldn't succeed in flying for another 50 years. (The two brothers flew in 1903.) A Parliamentary commission in the UK concluded that Thomas Edison's light-bulb was unworthy of the attention of practical or scientific men. In 1876, President Rutherford B Hayes tried out the new telephone gadget and, although impressed with it as a gadget, said he couldn't think why anyone would ever want to use one. Alexander Graham Bell tried to sell the idea of the telephone to Western Union but they weren't having any of it. And eminent British scientist Lord Kelvin dismissed radio as having no future.

In 1922, the editor of the *Daily Express* in London told an assistant to get rid of the man who had turned up at his offices announcing that he had just invented television. The man was John Logie Baird. A man who was thinking of investing in the Ford Motor Company was told that cars were just a novelty which wouldn't replace the horse. In 1943, the founder of the IBM said that he thought there was a world market for about five computers.

Even bright men have made daft statements. Albert Einstein said in 1932 that there wasn't the slightest indication that nuclear energy would ever be obtainable and useable.

Critics and reviewers in the world of literature have made enough mistakes to fill a book.

A Midsummer Night's Dream was described by Samuel Pepys as 'the most insipid, ridiculous play I ever saw'. When *Alice's Adventures in Wonderland* came out, a leading reviewer described the tale as 'stiff' and 'overwrought'. John Milton the poet was dismissed with the comment 'his fame is gone out like a candle…and his memory will always stink'. Charles Dickens was dismissed as unlikely to last. Herman Melville's classic *Moby Dick* was rejected as sad stuff, dull and dreary and ridiculous. A leading editor in the US told Kipling not to send in any more articles. An editor told Frederick Forsyth that his thriller *The Day of the Jackal* had no reader interest.

The experts in Hollywood haven't done much better. Marilyn Monroe was told to learn secretarial work or get married. *Gone with the Wind* was forecast to be the biggest flop in Hollywood history. A film studio executive rejected Burt Reynolds for having a chipped tooth and, in the same morning, rejected Clint Eastwood for talking too slowly. Critics dismissed *Annie Get Your Gun*, *Oklahoma* and *Grease* as having no future. The manager of the Grand Ole Opry told a young wannabe called Elvis Presley to go back to driving a truck. In 1962, a Decca Recording Company Executive turned down the Beatles. Six years earlier the same company had fired Buddy Holly, describing him as 'the biggest no-talent I ever worked with'.

It's the same everywhere you look. The experts make mistakes which now seem absurd but which were taken seriously because they were offered by experts.

Renoir was said to have no talent and told to give up painting. And a similar professional criticism was offered to Picasso, Degas and Cezanne.

In the world of justice and the law it has been shown that expert lawyers over-estimate their chances of winning in court. If both sides in a court case are asked who will win, each will say that its chances of winning are greater than 50%.

You might hope that experts in medicine would do better.

But they don't. Radiologists fail to diagnose lung disease in around a third of cases. Psychologists have been proved to be no better at making judgements (or offering advice) than individuals with no training. Indeed, hairdressers turned out to be more useful. One group of clinical psychologists claimed that their diagnoses were correct 90% of the time but in practice they were wrong more often than they were right. Research has shown that psychiatrists are worse than useless. And nurses and social workers are no better at making diagnoses or finding the correct treatment than the man or woman on the street.

Along with cancer and circulatory disease, doctors are now one of the three most important causes of death and injury. Incompetent or careless doctors cause a horrifying amount of death or injury. Many of the injuries and deaths among patients are caused by simple, straightforward incompetence rather than bad luck or unforeseen complications.

When doctors studied what happened to more than 30,000 patents admitted to acute care hospitals, they found that nearly 4% of them suffered unintended injuries in the course of their treatment and that 14% of the patients died of their injuries. Doctors kill vastly more innocent people than terrorists. Indeed, if terrorists killed a fraction of the number killed by doctors the world would be in a state of constant panic.

The medical literature is full of examples of doctor induced illness and death. At least a fifth of British patients who have slightly raised blood pressure are treated unnecessarily with drugs. At least a fifth of radiological examinations are clinically unhelpful. In the UK, doctors in casualty units kill at least one thousand patients a year.

Doctors (egged on by drug companies) often claim that it is thanks to them that we are all living longer these days and that drug companies and doctors have improved our general health. That's baloney. The evidence shows that there really hasn't been much change in life expectation in recent years. (After all, way back in Biblical times, ordinary folk were encouraged to expect a life-span of three score and ten.) Drug companies and doctors like to take all the credit for the alleged improvement, but the truth is that cleaner drinking water and better sewage facilities (introduced in the 19th century) resulted in a fall in infant mortality levels. And reducing infant mortality has made a tremendous difference to overall life expectancy figures. The general standards in most hospitals were low throughout the 18th and 19th centuries, and death rates were high. The Foundling Hospital in Dublin, for example, admitted 10,272 infants in the years from 1775 to 1796, and of these only forty-five survived. That sort of mortality rate among infants keeps life expectation figures low.

A study in Australia showed that 470,000 Australian men, women and children are admitted to hospital every year because they have been made ill by doctors. Figures in Europe are no better. One in six British hospital patients is in hospital and receiving treatment because he or she has been made ill by doctors. Around half of all the 'adverse events' associated with doctors are clearly and readily preventable and are usually a result of ignorance or incompetence or a mixture of both. The rest would be preventable with a little care and thought.

Everywhere you look there are scandals.

It was estimated in one medical publication that three quarters of surgeons were still using hernia repair techniques which were regarded internationally as obsolete. Once a surgeon has got a job, he is likely to stay set in his ways. Over the years the only thing that will change is that he will acquire an increasing number of prejudices and bad habits.

The regulators who are supposed to protect patients from dishonest or disreputable doctors seem generally unconcerned with things which really should concern them. When newspapers reported that a large drug company had been reprimanded by the industry's own 'watchdog' for paying doctors to switch patients from rival medicines to its own product there was no suggestion that the doctors involved might be subjected to professional discipline. These, remember, were doctors who had accepted bribes to change their patients' medication.

The astonishing truth is that most medical treatments recommended by experts are untried and have never been proved to be any good at all. Even drug treatments which are well-established have usually still not yet been properly thought out or evaluated. Prejudice and superstition are hardly a sound basis for good science.

Drugs are wildly over-prescribed, both by hospital doctors and by general practitioners. And doctors and hospitals are often appallingly and inexcusably slow. Doctors have always made mistakes and there have always been patients who have died as a result of medical ignorance or incompetence. But we have now reached the point where, on balance, many well-meaning doctors in general practice and many highly-trained, well-equipped specialists working in hospitals, do more harm than good. Through a mixture of ignorance and incompetence, doctors are killing more people than they are saving and they are causing more illness and more discomfort than they are alleviating.

It is true, of course, that doctors save thousands of lives by prescribing life-saving drugs such as antibiotics and by performing essential life-saving surgery on road accident victims. But the tragedy is that the good which doctors do is often far outweighed by the bad. What is even more worrying is the fact that the epidemic of iatrogenic disease (disease caused by doctors) which has scarred medical practice for decades has been steadily getting worse. Today most of us would, most of the time, be better off without a medical profession.

Thanks to recommendations from experts, doctors pay far too much attention to high technology equipment these days. Probably as a result, they are often frighteningly bad at making diagnoses. A study, published a few years ago showed that major disorders are not picked up in around four out of ten patients. When doctors compared post-mortem results with the patients' medical records, they discovered that out of 87 patients, only 17 patients were diagnosed completely correctly. Ten of the patients might have survived if the diagnosis had been more accurate. In 15 cases, major problems (such as heart attacks) were not detected.

Remember: one in six patients in hospital is there because he or she has been made ill by medical treatment.

It was in 1988 that I first warned about the danger of mammograms. My criticism was, of course, greeted with howls of outrage from the medical establishment. Back then I wrote: 'There are, of course, risks in having regular X-ray examinations. No one knows yet exactly what those risks are. We will probably find out in another ten or twenty years' time.'

In fact it was in 2006 that doctors finally issued a warning about mammograms, coming to precisely the conclusion I had warned about eighteen years earlier. Mammographic screening may help prevent breast cancer. But it may also cause breast cancer. Just how many women die because of the radiation they have received through mammography isn't known but it seems that the risks for younger women (women in their 30's for example) are higher than the risks for older women. (Radiation-induced cancer typically takes up to 20 years to develop, so for a woman in her 80's the risks of mammography are probably somewhere between slight and negligible.) According to some estimates, out of every 10,000 women who have mammograms from the age of 40 onwards, between two and four will develop radiation-induced breast cancer. One of them will die as a result of this. The precise figures are unknown and depend upon the quality and amount of the radiation, the skill of the technician and other factors – probably including the general health of the woman concerned.

Patients are frequently invited to their doctor's surgery for a screening test or a health check. In Britain, family doctors are paid huge bonuses if they perform routine health checks on their elderly patients. The experts agree that this is a 'good thing'.

The principle of screening is a simple one: the patient trots along to the doctor, and the doctor (for a chunky, great fee, of course) does tests which are designed to spot early signs of disease. The tests which are offered are done because the medical establishment has managed to convince bureaucrats that screening is worth paying for. Doctors are enthusiastic about screening because it's enormously profitable. And they're very lukewarm about encouraging their patients to follow healthier lifestyles because there is no money in it.

For decades now, just about every attempt to show that medical screening programmes save lives has proved that they are a waste of time, energy and money. Indeed, surveys have proved that, because of the risk of false positives, medical screening programmes do far more harm than good.

A major study of patients who'd had heart attacks showed that staying at home may be safer than going into hospital. The patients in the trial were allocated at random either to a hospital bed or to staying at home. The authors of the paper reported that the mortality rates for the two groups were similar. Whatever advantage patients might have had through going into hospital, and being surrounded by machines, doctors and nurses, was matched by the multiple hazards of going into hospital.

Before the industrial age, hospitals were built like cathedrals in order to lift the soul and ease the mind. Hospitals were decorated with carvings, works of art, flowers and perfumes. Modern hospitals, designed by experts, are built with no regard for the spirit, eye or soul. They are bare, more like prisons than temples, designed to concentrate the mind on pain, fear and death.

In the old days nurses were hired and trained to nurse. Aspiring nurses (mostly but not exclusively female) were inspired by the desire to tend and to heal. Nursing was a noble profession. Caring was the key word. The most powerful jobs in the profession were occupied by ward sisters and matrons – all of whom still had close, daily contact with patients.

Sadly, today's career structure, built on academic qualifications, means that nurses whose desire to nurse is accompanied by even the slightest ambition must quickly move up the ladder to a point where they spend very little time or, more probably no time at all, with patients.

The actual hands-on nursing is done by junior staff. This is, without a doubt, one of the reasons why modern hospitals are so bad.

In the United Kingdom the number of senior managers in hospitals has risen every year for decades. At the same time the number of nurses and cleaners keeps falling. There are more administrators in hospitals than there are beds, nurses or other practical staff. It is not surprising that staff spend much of their time filling in forms while the number of patients contracting serious, deadly infections continues to soar.

Moreover, thanks to the experts, hospitals are designed and built around the needs of the staff. To the architects who design hospitals, to the managers who run them, patients are, it seems, something of a nuisance, without whom everything would run far more smoothly.

Signs of administrators at work are everywhere. For example, it is the fashion these days to put carpets in hospital corridors. Naturally, this is dangerously unhealthy (since carpets are far more difficult to clean than other forms of flooring) but at least it means that administrators are not disturbed by the noise of patients being wheeled about.

A few decades ago patients were cared for in hospitals which were run by matrons and ward sisters – nurses who still knew how to turn a patient, make a bed and empty a bedpan. Many patients cannot, of course, remember how efficient hospitals were in those days and so, because they don't know what to expect or what to look for, they think they are being well looked after.

In many countries, doctors (both in general practice and in hospitals) are now working strictly limited hours. As a result, it is rare to see a doctor in a hospital at weekends. Patients are left lying in bed all weekend. No one, it seems, has heard of deep vein thromboses or pressure sores. You are between 8% and 26% more likely to die if you are admitted to hospital at the weekend than if you are admitted to hospital during the week.

Another problem is that you are more likely to catch a serious, life-threatening infection in hospital than anywhere else. The great danger is, of course, that you may catch an antibiotic resistant infection. Such infections were predictable (I predicted their development in 1977 in a book called *Paper Doctors)* and are avoidable (I explained how they could best be avoided in the same book) but are as a result of worsening hospital hygiene and the overuse of antibiotics. These resistant bugs are now a significant health threat in hospitals.

Hospital staff seem unconcerned at this, even though every incidence of MRSA infection is, like nearly all bed sores and most cases of deep vein thrombosis, straightforward evidence of poor nursing. Even medical records, pens and computer keyboards are now known to be infected with superbugs. Some hospitals have no changing facilities, and so nurses go home in their uniforms (taking bugs with them). Most hospitals don't launder uniforms and so nurses have to put their uniforms in with the family wash – usually at a temperature which will not destroy the bugs.

And then there are the operations.

Operations are potentially dangerous procedures and are best avoided whenever possible.

Surgical deaths in the United Kingdom alone number tens of thousands a year but nine out of ten operations are done to improve life rather than save life. This means that many of the patients who die as a result of surgery didn't *need* their operations. Little research has been done to find out if all those operations actually do improve the quality of life for the patients who have them.

Doctors have never taken much interest in preventive medicine or in how to help their patients stay healthy. This, I'm afraid, is because they have little or no financial interest in keeping their patients healthy. Except in China (where doctors were once paid only for as long as their patients stayed well) doctors have always earned their money out of diagnosing and curing illness. When you earn money out of making people healthy when they are ill, keeping them healthy makes no financial sense at all. Drug companies don't make money when people get better – they make money when people remain ill and need constant medication.

The drug companies, speaking to us via well-paid establishment experts, have persuaded doctors to encourage us to believe that when we are ill we must take something to rid ourselves of our symptoms. It's all about money.

It's because of this that doctors take very little interest in teaching people about healthy eating.

We were designed (or slowly evolved) for a very different type of diet to the one most of us eat today. We were designed for a diet based on fruits and vegetables, supplemented occasionally with a small amount of lean meat. We weren't designed to eat vast quantities of fatty meat, we weren't designed to drink milk taken from another animal (and meant for its young) and we weren't designed to eat grains.

Around 99.99% of our genetic material was formed when we were eating the sort of diet for which we were designed. But now most of us live on fatty meat, milky foods and cereals.

There were 100,000 generations of humans known as hunter-gatherers (living on fruits and vegetables they gathered and animals they occasionally managed to kill) and 500 generations dependent on agriculture (living on food grown on farms and animals reared in captivity). There have been just ten generations of humans since the onset of the industrial age and just two generations have grown up with highly processed fast, junk food. Knowing all this, it is hardly surprising that most of us ill most of the time.

And, of course, partly as a result of poor eating habits, obesity is now endemic in most Western countries. Type 2 diabetes (also known as maturity onset diabetes) is often a consequence of obesity. And yet most doctors do little or nothing either to help their patients to lose weight or to deal with Type 2 diabetes by managing their diet. In some countries, about a quarter of the people who have diabetes do not know that they have diabetes. When diabetes is diagnosed, the doctor's usual response is to reach for a prescription pad and prescribe one of the potentially hazardous drugs promoted for the purpose. In fact, most patients could control their diabetes (and protect themselves from health problems) by changing their diet (cutting out junk foods) and losing excess weight. But prescribing a pill is easier than giving advice. And taking a pill is easier than cutting down on chocolate bars.

Is it a coincidence that when gorillas are brought into captivity and fed on the sort of diet we think they should eat (not dissimilar, of course, from the sort of diet we eat ourselves) they too develop heart disease, ulcerative colitis and high cholesterol levels – problems they don't suffer from in the wild? Given the opportunity to become couch potatoes, baboons will jump at the idea. The Masai Mara National Reserve on the Serengeti Plains of Kenya had baboons who traditionally picked and chose their diet from everything available. But as the Park grew, it inevitably attracted tourists, hotels and rubbish. Within a few years of the first waste dump being formed, the baboons found that they could just lie around until the waste lorry arrived and then binge on high fat, high protein, high sugar leftovers. The baboons feeding like this grow faster, reach puberty earlier and weigh more. But their cholesterol levels shot up and they developed diabetes and chronic heart disease.

In North America the same thing happened to wild bears who hung around waste dumps and car parks in places such as the Yosemite National Park. They became obese and ill. And they also became mentally disturbed; showing signs of confusion and becoming increasingly violent.

Is it coincidence that the hunter-gatherer societies which still exist in the world's few wild, remote areas have far less cancer, heart disease, diabetes and osteoporosis? They may die falling from trees or being eaten by wild animals but they don't die from the sort of diseases which cripple and kill us. Time and time again anthropologists have observed that as native societies abandon their traditional hunter-gatherer lifestyle, so their health deteriorates.

Today, we are like captive cows and sheep, falling ill because we can no longer choose a varied diet but must rely on what the farmers and the supermarkets choose to offer us.

If doctors told their patients the truth about food, most of the world's drug companies would virtually disappear within months.

12

The market for heart drugs, high blood pressure drugs, anti-cancer drugs and so on would fall through the floor. Drug companies would be struggling along side-by-side with the buggy whip manufacturers.

And yet the advice about nutrition given to patients by doctors, nurses, nutritionists and dieticians is often appalling and frequently lethal. The food served in hospitals (where people are, it can safely be assumed, at their weakest and at their greatest need of wholesome, nutritious food) is almost universally inedible and customarily harmful to the patient. The food produced for patients is nothing more than unwholesome stodge, full of calories and fat and devoid of vitamins.

Finally, there is clear evidence to show that how much food you eat is just as important as what you eat. Eating less can lead to a longer life.

A team from the Louisiana State University in the USA monitored a group of 48 overweight men and women aged between 25 and 50 years. A quarter of them were put on a diet containing 25% fewer calories than they would be expected to eat for their age and weight. Another quarter had their calorie intake reduced by 12.5% and was also put on a strict exercise regime. A third group stuck to a very strict diet of just 890 calories a day. Finally, the last group was placed on a diet which would enable them to maintain their weight.

The results showed that the volunteers on the fewest calories lost, on average, 14% of their body weight during the six months. The other calorie-restricted dieters lost 10% of their body weight. All the volunteers who cut down their calories showed a fall in their average body temperature and showed reduced fasting insulin levels – both figures which are linked to longevity. The rate at which their DNA decayed also slowed. This is important because decaying DNA increases the chances of mutations and degenerative diseases developing, and producing problems such as cancer.

Other research has shown that people who eat less also have healthier hearts.

Researchers believe that cutting calories reduces the production of free radicals, the toxic particles which are difficult for the body to get rid of. The message is simple: eat less, live longer.

If you eat like a bird you'll live as long as an elephant.

So why don't doctors and dieticians warn patients of this?

The answer, I'm afraid, is frighteningly simple and can be summed up in a question.

Where's the profit?

Improving diets might save lives, but it wouldn't help the drug companies increase their profits.

Most doctors are unquestioning – too frightened to upset the establishment. Asking uncomfortable questions can ruin a doctor's career. And medical journalists are just as useless. Most have very little formal medical training, they don't know what to look for, they not infrequently receive payments from drug companies and they hardly ever have the courage to take on the establishment. Far too many so-called medical and health journalists are wimpy incompetents who won't print or broadcast anything which might damage their cosy relationships with the medical establishment and the international pharmaceutical industry.

The doctors and nurses who do know the truth don't dare talk about it. And, sadly, most doctors and nurses don't bother to search out the facts. They just recite what they're told by the drug companies, prescribe vast quantities of pills, recommend huge numbers of vaccinations (because that is what they are told to do) and carefully avoid seeking or sharing out the truth.

There are fashions in medicine just as much as there are fashions in clothes. The difference is that whereas badly conceived fashions in clothes are only likely to embarrass you, ill-conceived fashions in medicine may kill you. The fashions in medicine have, by and large, as much scientific validity as the fashions in the clothes industry.

The most obvious fashions in medicine relate to treatments. For example, a couple of centuries ago, enemas, purges and bleedings were all the rage. In 17th century France, Louis XIII had 212 enemas, 215 purges and 47 bleedings in a single year. The Canon of Troyes is reputed to have had a total of 2,190 enemas in a two year period; how he found time to do anything else is difficult to imagine. By the mid-19th century, enemas were a little last year's style and bleeding was the in-thing. There was even a posh word for it – doctors who were about to remove blood from their patients would say that they were going to phlebotomize them. Patients would totter into their doctor's surgery, sit down, tuck up their sleeves and ask the doctor to 'draw me a pint of blood'. Bleeding was the universal cure, recommended for most symptoms and ailments. 'Feeling a little under the weather? A little light bleeding should soon put you to rights.' 'Constant headaches? We'll soon have that sorted for you, sir. Just roll up your sleeve.' 'Bit of trouble down below, madam? Not to worry. Hold your arm out.'

A little later, in the nineteenth century, doctors put their lancets away and started recommending alcohol as the new panacea. Brandy was the favoured remedy in the doctor's pharmacopoeia. People took it for almost everything. And when patients developed delirium tremens, the recommended treatment was more alcohol. If things got so bad that the brandy didn't work, doctors added a little opium. Those were the days to be ill. Hypochondriacs must have had a wonderful time.

In the years from the 1930s onwards, removing tonsils became the fashionable treatment. Tonsils were removed from between a half and three-quarters of all children in the 1930s. This often useless and unnecessary, and always potentially hazardous, operation is less commonly performed these days but in the 1970s, over a million such operations were done every year in Britain alone. Doctors used to rip out tonsils on the kitchen table. Between 200 and 300 deaths a year were caused by the operation. One suspects that few, if any, of those unfortunate children would have died from tonsillitis.

Diseases go in cycles too.

One year everyone will be suffering from asthma. It will be the disease of the moment just as the mini skirt or ripped jeans may drift mysteriously in and out of fashion. Another year arthritis will be the fashionable disease as a drug company persuades journalists to write articles extolling the virtues (and disguising the vices) of its latest product. The cycle is a relatively simple one. The drug company with a new and profitable product to sell (usually designed for some long-term – and therefore immensely profitable – disorder) will send teams of well-trained representatives around to talk to family physicians, give them presents and take them out for expensive luncheons. The sales representatives will be equipped with information showing that the disorder in question is rapidly reaching epidemic proportions, lists of warning symptoms for the doctor to watch out for and information about the drug company's new solution to the problem. Because the product will be new to the market, there will probably be very little evidence available about

15

side effects and the sales representative will be accurately able to describe the drug as extremely 'safe'.

And the number of prescriptions being written for the new wonder product will soon rocket – pushing up drug company profits dramatically.

Then, a year or so later, patients and doctors alike will become aware of the many side effects associated with the new alleged wonder product and prescribing levels will fall. It is then the turn of some other product and some other disease to take the limelight and some other drug company to enjoy a dramatic boost in its profits.

For years now surgeons have been performing unnecessary operations; operations which have done far more harm than good. It is, of course, difficult to be precise about the number of unnecessary operations but in America, researchers have concluded that in an average sort of year, surgeons working in American hospitals now perform 7.5 million unnecessary surgical procedures, resulting in 37,136 unnecessary deaths and a cost running into hundreds of billions of dollars. One Congressional Committee in the US found that 17.6% of recommendations for surgery were not necessary.

Nothing illustrates the uselessness (and danger) of elective surgery more completely than heart surgery. In America, having had at least one coronary artery bypass operation is now as much a sign of success as ownership of a Mercedes limousine. And the operation is growing in popularity around the rest of the world. In Britain around 10% of the people who have had heart attacks end up having heart bypass operations.

Many surgeons claim that surgery for heart disease is not elective but vital. But the evidence shows that most of the surgery performed for the treatment of heart disease is entirely unnecessary. Back in 1988 (in a now out of print book called *The Health Scandal)* I reported that coronary artery bypass surgery (the commonest procedure performed in cardiac surgery) had been in use for nearly thirty years without anyone trying to find out how patients' everyday lives were affected by the operation. The experts just 'knew' it was a good thing.

When a survey was eventually done, it was found that whereas nearly half of the patients who had the operation had been working right up to the time of surgery, three months after the operation only just over a third of the men were working. And a year after the operation, nearly half the patients were still not working. In other words, the operation had little positive effect on patients' lives but did put a good many out of action for some time. There were, of course, a number of patients who died as a result of surgical complications.

And what makes the medical profession's enthusiasm for coronary artery surgery even more bizarre is the fact that research done by Dr Dean Ornish has shown that patients who have symptoms of heart disease often don't need surgery at all but stand a better chance of recovering if they are put on a regime which includes a vegan diet, gentle exercise and relaxation.

The vast majority of medical journalists, who might be expected to criticise unnecessary medical procedures which put patients' lives at risk, know little or nothing of medical matters and are too much in awe of the medical establishment (and its most vocal experts) to offer any sort of criticism.

Psychiatrists and psychologists are also eager to create fashionable new bandwagons too. It is now possible to be clinically afraid of over 500 different things, for that is the astonishing number of phobias which have been officially recognised. In addition to traditional phobias such as claustrophobia, patients can now suffer from kakorrhaphiophobia (a fear of defeat), apeirophobia (a fear of infinity), chrometophobia (a fear of money) and hippopotomonstros-esquippedaliphobia (a fear of long words). It's difficult to tell when the experts are being serious and when they're having us on these days. (But these *are* real.)

There is no doubt that drug companies exaggerate mild problems in order to boost their profits, and they devise and then promote non-existent diseases in order to create fashionable new markets for their drugs. They use well-paid experts to promote the newly invented diseases.

In 1991, one in ten hospital deaths was followed by a post mortem. In 2004, the figure had fallen to 1 in 40. Today, post mortems are almost a rarity. When fewer post mortems are performed, doctors are less likely to be embarrassed by evidence showing that they made a big mistake. Doctors are also, of course, unlikely to learn anything if they never know how wrong they were.

A former Director General of the World Health Organisation, some years ago, startled the medical establishment by stating that:

'the major and most expensive part of medical knowledge as applied today appears to be more for the satisfaction of the health professions than for the benefit of the consumers of health care'. The evidence certainly supports that view.

Consider what happens when doctors go on strike and leave patients to cope without professional medical help. You might imagine that people would be dying like flies in autumn. Not a bit of it. When doctors in Israel went on strike for a month, admissions to hospital dropped by eighty five per cent, with only the most urgent cases being admitted, but despite this the death rate in Israel dropped by fifty per cent – the largest drop since the previous doctors' strike twenty years earlier – to its lowest ever recorded level. Much the same thing has happened wherever doctors have gone on strike.

A report published in the *Journal of the Royal Society of Medicine* concluded that many hospital patients who suffer heart attacks die during the 'confused and disorganised charades' of attempts to save them because hospital doctors do not know how to give emergency resuscitation. Only rarely does real life match the efficiency (and success) of the television emergency ward.

Even more worrying was an editorial published in the *British Medical Journal* which stated that: 'only one per cent of the articles in medical journals are scientifically sound' and that 'only about fifteen per cent of medical interventions are supported by solid scientific evidence'. In other words the majority of treatments are completely untried and when a doctor writes out a prescription or sticks a knife into a patient, neither he nor anyone else has much of an idea about what will happen next.

Today, television and radio programmes always present experts as though their word is beyond discussion. Newspapers do the same, quoting experts as though they are bringing us solid evidence that the rest of us could never find without them.

It is frighteningly easy to become an 'expert'. When I was in my 20s and newly qualified, I was regularly described as a 'world famous expert' or a 'leading expert' whenever I was quoted in the media. At least I was only ever giving my opinion based on the facts which were available – I have never been paid or otherwise bribed to offer an opinion or a particular point of view.

There is a certain amount of irony in the fact that now I am much older, and I hope wiser and better informed, I am never invited to give my opinion on TV or radio shows or for the press. The mainstream media prefers its experts to stick to the official and accepted line on whatever topic is under discussion. What viewers, listeners and readers don't know is that many so-called experts have been bought and paid for, and when they open their mouths they are merely saying what they've been told to say by their employers. The drug industry has an army of doctors who will say whatever they are required to say – in return for a large cheque, a holiday abroad or a new television set. Special agencies offer these so-called experts to media groups who are looking for someone who can provide an apparently expert view. Television reporters, radio presenters and newspaper journalists like the fact that these experts work free of charge because they are paid by their sponsors. The 'experts' are known as 'rent a quote experts'.

When I was young, and earning a living in the media, I always expected to be paid a fee but after a while I found that I couldn't compete with the many doctors who were prepared to work without a fee or even expenses because they were paid by a drug company. When I wrote a syndicated newspaper column, the agency selling the column suddenly found that a few newspapers were cancelling the column. The editors of those papers explained that they'd been offered a free column as a replacement for mine. The writers of the free column were being paid, of course, but they were being paid by drug companies or government departments.

It should be clear by now that experts have screwed up in almost every area of life, and medical experts have been particularly adept at screwing up.

But that's only part of the problem with so-called experts.

The other part of the problem (and the subject of this book) is the way that the experts within the medical establishment (often controlled by lobbyists working for a variety of industries – including most notably the pharmaceutical industry) frequently suppress and crush important and original work that could save lives and improve the health of patients around the world.

This isn't a new phenomenon – it's been happening for centuries.

The medical establishment will always take decisions on health matters which benefit industry, government and the medical profession, rather than patients. And the Government will always take decisions on health matters which benefit the State and the pharmaceutical industry rather than individual patients.

Responsibility has been separated from authority with disastrous consequences for patients.

There is something uncivilised and inhuman about a health system, designed by experts and reliant on experts, in which patients with suspected cancer must wait weeks, months or years to see a specialist, wait weeks or months to be diagnosed and then wait weeks or months or years to be treated – hoping that they won't die on one of the waiting lists.

Finally, look at the way that experts have allowed our environment and our food to be poisoned by chemical companies, farmers and others involved in 'serving' our communities.

Poisons in our environment are now one of the most significant modern causes of illness in general and of cancer in particular. As a result of the contaminants in our food, drinking water and the air we breathe, human breast milk contains so many chemical contaminants that it couldn't possibly be sold as safe for human consumption. And human bodies contain so many chemicals (some consumed in additive and pesticide contaminated food and some acquired accidentally from our polluted environment) that a human steak would never be passed fit for consumption by cannibals.

Children's bodies are routinely contaminated with scores of potentially hazardous chemicals. The susceptibility of the young body, and the wide availability of toxic chemicals in the surroundings in which children live, mean that those as young as nine-years-old have far more toxic substances in their bodies than their grandparents ever had.

Television sets and plastic toys, deodorants and household cleansers are all sources of poisons as, of course, are the pesticides we use in our garden and the pesticides farmers use on our food.

Some carcinogenic industrial chemicals which have been banned can still be found in the environment. Back in 1930, just one million tons of man-made chemicals were produced globally each year. Today, the chemical companies produce hundreds of millions of tons of man-made chemicals a year.

When researchers tested ordinary citizens, they found that of 104 substances for which they had tested, 80 were present in human beings. These tests are often repeated – with much the same results.

Chemicals are in our air, our water and our food. The chemicals found in the average human body can cause liver cancer, damage to the developing brain, premature birth, genital abnormalities, bladder cancer, kidney damage, asthma, skin disorders, hormone disruption, and a higher risk of miscarriage.

There is not enough safety information available about nearly 90% of the 2,500 chemicals which manufacturers regularly use in large quantities, to enable scientists or doctors to do a basic safety assessment.

When chemicals are tested they are tested on animals. If the tests show that a chemical kills animals, the test will be ignored on the grounds that animals are so different to humans that the results are irrelevant, and manufacturers will be allowed to use the chemical as much as they like. Drug companies follow the same 'we can't lose' trickery when testing drugs.

There is no doubt at all that many of the chemicals widely used in the preparation of food, the feeding of animals and the manufacture of a wide variety of goods are carcinogenic.

The experts know all this, of course, but they do nothing to prevent the pollution, or to deal with it because to do so would inconvenience their paymasters.

Then there is the scandal of our drinking water.

In towns and cities, drinking water is often taken from rivers. But sewage firms dump their untreated waste into the same rivers. The real problem is the fact that they can't remove drug residues from the human waste which is discharged into the rivers. The result is that when you turn on your tap you get bits of old contraceptive pill, antibiotic and tranquilliser in your sparkling glass of apparently clean drinking water. You can't see the drug residues, of course. And the water companies can't get them out.

Governments have, of course, made things worse by adding fluoride to drinking water supplies. The theory is that if people drink water dosed with fluoride they will be less likely to suffer from dental decay. In practice, fluoride is a potentially hazardous substance and this practice is fraught with danger. Adding fluoride to the water is, however, encouraged by politicians because their ill-informed experts claim that although it probably damages the health of some citizens they claim it may help cut the nation's dental bill.

As part of a school science project, a 12-year-old American girl collected ice samples from five restaurants. She also collected loo water samples from the same restaurants. She had all the samples tested for bacteria. In several cases, the ice from the restaurants contained e.coli bacteria and was dirtier than the water taken from the loo bowls. How did the bugs get into the ice?

Probably because the ice-making machines hadn't been cleaned and because the restaurant staff had used hands which hadn't been washed to scoop up the ice.

The moral is a simple one: you should avoid ice in bars and restaurants.

Doctors exist only for two reasons: to look after people who have acquired a disease, and to prevent healthy people from falling ill. That's it. The rest is unimportant.

But today's medical profession has been bribed by drug companies, bullied by, and overwhelmed by bureaucrats and social workers, and forced by politicians to abandon most of their ethical principles (including, for example, the traditional principle of confidentiality). Through the weakness of their leaders, doctors have been turned into ethically impoverished mercenaries.

Principles should be indigestible but the modern medical profession has swallowed its principles without hesitation or regret.

It is, perhaps, hardly surprising that many doctors now hate their jobs and regard them as little more than a way of making money. Many doctors would prefer to do something else for a living – if they could find something as lucrative. Thanks largely to the activities of dishonest 'experts', vocation has been abandoned and replaced by expediency.

Medicine used to be a proud and independent profession. Sadly, much of the modern medical profession is now little more than a marketing arm for the pharmaceutical industry and a snitch service for the Government. And things are likely to get worse rather than better unless and until we force governments and doctors to recognise that people must come first.

In the second part of this monograph I'm going to give examples of how, why and when the medical establishment suppressed significant new ideas and scientific breakthroughs simply because they were seen as a threat to the status quo, or because they were regarded as offering an unwelcome criticism of the medical establishment.

Part Two
Medical Heretics and Conspiracy Theorists

Uncomfortable truths have always attracted abuse, ridicule and persecution and those who dare to speak out against the establishment have always been regarded as dangerous heretics. Governments and their hacks have always accused the truth-tellers of their own faults. The iconoclast has never been a welcome figure in any age. Original thinkers, daring to question the establishment, are still being demonised, 'de-platformed' and cancelled by a modern culture which may appear to offer more freedom than ever but which, in reality, is just as constrained, as restrictive and as destructive as anything in history. The truth is not always agreeable, acceptable or convenient to those in charge.

Confucius, the Chinese philosopher, was dismissed by his political masters and his books were burned. Those who didn't burn his books within 30 days were branded and condemned to forced labour. Socrates was accused of corrupting the youth of Athens, arrested for being an evildoer and 'a person showing curiosity, searching into things under the earth and above the heaven and teaching all this to others'. He was condemned to death. Dante, the Italian poet, was banished from Florence and condemned to be burnt at the stake if ever captured. After they had failed to silence him with threats and bribes, the authorities excommunicated Spinoza in Amsterdam because he refused to toe the party line, refused to think what other people told him he must think and insisted on maintaining his intellectual independence. He and his work were denounced as 'forged in Hell'.

Governments once burned original thinkers at the stake for believing that the earth went round the sun. There may not be much burning at the stake going on these days but original thinkers are destroyed by being described as 'conspiracy theorists' or, for absolutely no solid reason at all, and with no supporting evidence for the slur, they are labelled 'discredited'.

So, for example, the controlled editors of a fake encyclopaedia called Wikipedia are, if they are notable for anything, notable for their enthusiasm for replacing inconvenient truths with commercially or politically acceptable lies.

Doctors or scientists who even dare to question the officially accepted line on the use of drugs or vaccines (which will usually be the line preferred by the pharmaceutical industry) are likely to find themselves fired or to discover that their grant applications are denied. The licensing authorities may remove the licenses or registration of doctors who even dare to question the officially approved line of thinking. Even threatening doctors with the loss of their livelihood is enough to silence many. It is now increasingly common in Europe, America and Australasia for doctors who voice views which question drug industry research to be told that they must be suffering from mental illness and to be offered medical help for their 'mental illness'. This was, of course, a technique commonly used in the USSR to silence dissidents.

Charles Darwin didn't fare terribly well, either. After Darwin published his book *On the Origin of Species* many of the reviews weren't exactly encouraging. Professor Samuel Haughton of Dublin claimed that 'all that was new...was false, and what was true was old'. The ghost of Darwin may be amused by the fact that Haughton is now largely remembered only for his criticism of Darwin. Modern critics may be amused by the fact that Haughton was an early mathematical modeller and, therefore, one of the first in a long line of similarly labelled incompetents.

Not surprisingly, exactly the same thing has happened in the world of medicine where the establishment has always oppressed original thinkers, suppressed new ideas, rejected almost anything likely to help patients and demonised those physicians daring to suggest that the traditional way of doing something might be wrong.

This monograph explains how innovative doctors and scientists were sneered at by the medical establishment and how their work was suppressed, in some cases for centuries. I will detail some of the doctors who fought the medical establishment and (eventually) won.

The establishment has always opposed good, original ideas which threaten the status quo. And in the last century or so, the medical establishment has always done everything it could to protect the international pharmaceutical industry. This part of this book is about

25

doctors who changed things for the good – despite being sneered at, suppressed, oppressed, demonised and threatened. Many of the most significant discoveries in medicine were suppressed and truths distorted simply to satisfy the medical establishment.

The truth is that original thinkers and people who do not fit neatly into the scheme of things have never gone down well and, sadly, many of the greatest men (and occasionally women) in medicine have died ignored, forgotten or in disgrace.

So, for example, it is not difficult to argue that Dr John Snow, the English general practitioner who practised in the 19th century and who led the way in two medical specialities (anaesthesiology and epidemiology) did more for health care than all the world's drug companies put together. And yet he is largely forgotten: he received no honours, during life or post mortem and there is no statue to him. The only remembrance is the public house on the corner of what used to be Broad Street, which is named after him. Even the name of the street, which is in London's Soho district, was changed from Broad Street to Broadwick Street by councillors and officials with no sense of history.

A couple of centuries earlier, Aureolus Philippus Theophrastus Bombastus von Hohenheim (known to his chums as Paracelsus) made himself enemies all over Europe because he tried to revolutionise medicine in the sixteenth century. Paracelsus was the greatest influence on medical thinking since Hippocrates but the establishment regarded him as a trouble-maker and, indeed, large parts of the medical establishment still regard him with distaste.

I've written short essays about some of the most innovative thinkers in medicine – all of whom suffered to some extent or another at the hands of the medical establishment. Some were treated cruelly, some were professionally ruined and some were simply ignored or ostracised.

Andreas Vesalius (1514-1564)

Andreas Vesalius, one of the great pioneers of the Renaissance pioneers, was born in 1514 at about the time that Paracelsus embarked on his travels. Vesalius, a Belgian, achieved contemporary notoriety and eternal fame as the author of the first textbook of human anatomy, published in 1543 and called *De Humanis Corporis Fabrica*. The end of the fifteenth century and the beginning of the sixteenth century in Europe had seen a tremendous upsurge in interest in human anatomy, and with increasing numbers of students and scholars able to study copies of the ancient texts produced by such men as Galen, it was inevitable that the infallibility of these ideas was questioned. Once it was recognised that Galen could be wrong, many students began to offer original observations and theories.

(Galen was a Greek physician who worked with the gladiators in Rome. His theories and writings influenced medical practice for more than a thousand years. He was a clever physician and imaginative writer who used herbs as medicines and made much progress in this area. Sadly, his views on human anatomy were largely wrong and misleading. It wasn't his fault but Galen's errors stifled progress in medicine for a long time.)

The inaccuracy of Galen's anatomical notes was made more obvious by the fact that, for the first time in centuries, human anatomy could be studied by practical dissection, now that the influence of the Church had declined. As a result, artists and students of medicine were all anxious to dissect, study and draw human cadavers.

Leonardo da Vinci was one of the many multi-talented Renaissance men whose interests included anatomy. Contemporaries such as Michelangelo, Raphael and Durer all performed their own dissections and made drawings as they struggled to improve their knowledge of human anatomy.

Da Vinci had planned to publish a textbook of anatomical drawings, but Andreas Vesalius was the first to do so. His frank rejection of many of Galen's anatomical claims earned him considerable disapproval, since leaders of the medical establishment still firmly believed that Galen could not be wrong, even if the evidence proved otherwise.

For more than a thousand years, Galen had been considered beyond criticism, and his reputation was not to be easily overthrown.

Poor Vesalius was unable to cope with the outcry his researches in anatomy produced. He burnt his remaining manuscripts, abandoned the study of anatomy and took a job as court physician to Charles V in Madrid.

But those who attacked him could not change the fact that Vesalius's book had revealed the fallibility of the ancient texts, and the study of anatomy continued in art centres and medical schools all over Europe.

Sadly, it wasn't until the end of the 18th century and beginning of the 19th that doctors really began to understand human anatomy.

At the beginning of the 16th century, surgery was almost completely in the hands of uneducated wanderers who could be just as happy gelding a man's pig or cutting his hair as he would be amputating his leg. The barber-surgeons were indeed barbers, who supplemented their income from work with the scissors by working with the knife.

However, once it became clear that anatomical understanding could make the preparation and execution of surgical operations more of a scientific endeavour than an exercise in butchery, more educated men began to take up the profession. As the 16th century got under way, physicians in France and England at last acknowledged surgeons as professional colleagues.

Gradually, the dissection of human cadavers became an essential part of medical training, not only for the student anatomist but also for the clinician anxious to learn more about the pathology of human disorders. However, while, in many parts of Europe, there was a plentiful supply of corpses for doctors to dissect, the ready availability of human material was not universal.

Until 1751, in Britain the only legally available corpses were the four criminals annually allocated to the Barber Surgeons' Company in London. After 1751, the law was changed to make the corpses of all executed criminals available to anatomists, but the old-fashioned habit of gibbeting corpses meant that there was still a shortage. This led to the growth of a night-time industry dedicated to supplying the medical profession with corpses.

One of the first men to link anatomy with clinical science was the Edinburgh physician Robert Knox, whose attractive lecturing style kept the lecture theatre full – he is said to have had a regular class of over five hundred students. Unfortunately there was a shortage of cadavers at that time in Edinburgh, and the unhappy Knox became involved in one of the great medical scandals of the century.

Bodies were obtained by people like Knox in a number of ways from a variety of sources. Poor people sometimes sold the bodies of their dying relatives, and corpses were sometimes removed from coffins by unscrupulous undertakers, who buried an earth-filled coffin and sold the corpse. A more dramatic method of obtaining fresh corpses was simply to dig them up. It is said that in Britain in the 1820s, a total of some two hundred men were busy digging up bodies and removing them from churchyards. Some of these early 'resurrectionists' were undoubtedly medical students or anatomy lecturers looking for material for themselves, but many were common criminals who would steal anything for a good price. Corpse-stealing had been an offence since 1788 but relatively few people were caught and, when they were, sentences were usually light.

There was, of course, one way to obtain corpses for dissection which did not involve skulking around in churchyards at the dead of night. Murder was the technique favoured by two Irishmen, Burke and Hare, in 1827. They began their careers on the fringe of medicine by selling the body of a dead lodger which was about to be carted away for a pauper's funeral. Encouraged by the ease with which they made this sale, the two unemployed men then suffocated two more lodgers who seemed ill and apparently likely to die. Business continued to be profitable, and eventually Burke and Hare took their total number of victims to sixteen. All these bodies were happily bought by Dr Knox and his assistants.

When the two men were eventually caught, Hare turned King's evidence and, as a result, was allowed to leave Edinburgh, while Burke was hanged and later dissected by Professor Alexander Monro, who held the chair of anatomy at Edinburgh University. The unhappy Knox was virtually ruined by the scandal, since the body of one of the victims was found in his private dissecting room. The medical profession, which contained many men as guilty as Knox, managed to keep clear of the scandal. The Burke and Hare murders resulted in the passing of an Anatomy Act in 1832 which ruled that all unclaimed dead bodies should go to the medical schools for dissection.

It had taken nearly 300 years for the work of Vesalius to have a real impact on medical practice.

Roger Bacon (1214-1294)

Roger Bacon, who lived from 1214 to 1298, was an original thinker at a time when original thinking was rare and dangerous to your health. Even at Salerno, Bologna, Padua, Montpellier and the other centres of academic excellence, most work was confined to the study and intellectual dissection of the ancient Greek texts. Bacon was a Franciscan monk who had been well educated both as a philosopher and as a natural scientist, and it was his work that made the Paris medical school famous.

Bacon was one of the first scientists to insist that chemicals could be used medicinally and that alchemy had a role to play in human pharmacology, Bacon found himself battling against the entire establishment. Galen had favoured herbal medicines, and the medical establishment revered the works of Galen. The Church strongly objected to Bacon's theories because it seemed dangerously sacrilegious for a monk to suggest that the Will of God could be influenced with the aid of a handful of chemicals.

Not that Bacon confined himself to the study of drugs. He is said to have invented a telescope, a microscope and the first spectacles, and prophesied powered flight and underwater exploration. He performed a great many original scientific experiments. All this made him desperately unpopular with almost all sectors of established thought, and Bacon became the first of the scientific martyrs who were to litter the history of the Renaissance.

Paracelsus (Aureolus Theophrastus Bombastus von Hohenheim) (1493-1541)

The history of medicine is richly peppered with fascinating, colourful and often controversial characters. The Renaissance was an excellent time for men who were more interested in scientific truth than in acknowledged prejudices, and the first half of the sixteenth century was a time of much controversy and original thinking.

One of the most controversial, and undoubtedly one of the most colourful characters in medical history, was a man called Paracelsus who may well have contributed as much as any other individual in the history of medical science to modern medical progress.

Paracelsus, was christened Aureolus Theophrastus Bombastus von Hohenheim when he was born in 1493. Not surprisingly, perhaps, he was better known as Paracelsus. Born in Switzerland, Paracelsus, who died just 48 years later in 1541, tore into the precepts of established medical thinking with all the zeal of an inspired missionary. He revolutionised medical thinking throughout Europe.

The most revealing of the many stories about Paracelsus reports him as having claimed to have learned more from his contact with witches and midwives than from a study of the ancient and previously well respected texts of such classical authors as Galen.

Paracelsus was one of the first practitioners to believe that it was possible to learn by experience and personal study. He travelled widely in the search for useful medical information. He went to Spain, Portugal, France, Italy, Germany, Scandinavia, Egypt, Arabia, Palestine, Russia, Poland, Turkey, Holland and England to study, work and meet like-minded people. He wrote books, lectured, practised medicine and argued in Montpellier, Padua, Bologna, Basle, Vienna, Tubingen, Wittenberg, Leipzig, Heidelberg and Cologne – almost all the major medical centres of Europe. No idea or theory was too bizarre for his attention and no concept or belief too sacred to be rejected. He studied alchemy, astrology and herbal medicine in his search for information.

Paracelsus believed that a doctor's job was to understand the causes and symptoms of different diseases and to prescribe specific solutions where appropriate. He also believed in the importance of preventing disease and was one of the first members of the medical profession to recognise that there is often an association between a man's employment and his physical condition.

Paracelsus's writings make formidable reading, and he was an important figure in Renaissance medicine. He was the first man to associate mining with certain chest diseases, to link cretinism and goitres with certain alpine areas, to use mercury in the treatment of syphilis, to advocate allowing wounds to drain instead of smothering them with layers of dried dung, and to argue that some foods contained poisons which had a deleterious effect on the human body.

But all these important advances seem almost irrelevant when put alongside his philosophical contributions and his effect on the attitude of the men studying medicine in the sixteenth century.

Paracelsus was really the first 'people's doctor', and he proudly claimed that he pleased only the sick and not the medical profession.

He bombarded medical students and scholars with a seemingly endless selection of almost blasphemous assertions, which encouraged them to think for themselves and to reject the previously unquestioned preachings of such authorities as Galen.

He seems at times to have enjoyed humiliating the establishment, as for example when he welcomed barber-surgeons as well as official medical students to his lectures at Basle, but there is little doubt that this extraordinary man was the father of modern medicine and the sixteenth century equivalent of Hippocrates.

Inevitably, Paracelsus was the object of much derision and opposition and he was constantly on the move around Europe – keeping ahead of his critics.

Even today, Paracelsus is still derided by members of the medical establishment who criticise the cures he offered as being of little real value but in doing so fail to understand that Paracelsus's contribution to the development of medical science lay not in the introduction of specific cures (it is hardly realistic to expect him to have single-handedly introduced a comprehensive medical pharmacopeia) but in introducing elements of real science into medicine, for fathering scientific enquiry, for replacing magic and old wives tales with a fundamental enthusiasm for rational processes and for breaking with medical traditions which were built on centuries old beliefs which had held medicine in a backwater for over a thousand years.

It is entirely to his credit that Paracelsus was driven from Switzerland by orthodox physicians who preferred to remain in the past and who refused to allow anyone even to question their outdated, dangerous methods of practice.

Paracelsus died in exile in Salzburg because he asked questions and because he offered revolutionary solutions to age old problems.

Sadly, little or nothing has changed.

Girolamo Fracastorio (1478-1553), Antonj van Leeuwenhoek (1632-1723), William Petty (1623-1687)

During the Renaissance many attempts were made to explain the precise nature of infectious diseases. The most astonishing attempt was the work of Hieronymus Fracastorio, a Veronese nobleman who, in 1541, published a book entitled *De Contagione*.

Fracastorio, whose foresight stands out even among the extraordinary intellectual explosions of the sixteenth century, suggested that contagious diseases were disseminated by small particles of matter which were able to multiply rapidly and which could be spread through the air, by simple, direct contact or from one individual to another through infected clothing.

Fracastorio's valuable book, the basis of the modern germ theory, was virtually ignored at the time because there was no real evidence to support the theory.

It was almost another 150 years before the remarkable microscopist Antonie van Leeuwenhoek described bacteria for the first time. Leeuwenhoek's day job (or jobs) was as a draper and city hall janitor in Delft. In his spare time he had ground more than four hundred lenses and built more than two hundred microscopes.

Sadly, neither Fracastorius nor Leeuwenhoek had any impact on death rates and no progress was made in the treatment of infection until the 19th century in England.

Despite their discoveries, epidemics continued to affect Europe, and the mortality rate from infectious diseases was still as great in the seventeenth century as it had been in the less enlightened Middle Ages. The plague hit Italy in 1630 and killed 80,000 in Milan alone. In the Venetian Republic over half a million are said to have died. In Moscow in 1603 more than 120,000 succumbed, in 1679 Vienna lost 70,000, and in Prague in 1681 83,000 died.

Throughout the century the plague came and went, affecting France, Italy, Denmark, Germany, Sweden, Switzerland, Spain, the

Netherlands and England. Individual attacks of plague were often followed by economic disaster and famine. London was affected in 1624 when 41,000 were killed, in 1635 when another 10,000 died and finally in 1664 when the total number of dead was nearly 70,000.

Europe is still littered with statues and local customs originally created by citizens anxious to give thanks for having avoided the plague. In the English county of Derbyshire, for example, where the villagers of Eyam contracted the plague through a parcel of clothes sent from London, many modern villagers still dress and deck their wells with flowers each year. The wells enabled the individual villages to remain tightly knit, closed communities and therefore helped to prevent the spread of the plague.

Attempts to prevent the plague spreading and to deal with those suffering from the disease varied from town to town and from country to country. Since no one knew exactly what caused the plague or helped it to spread, attempts to control it were not always devoid of hysteria and superstition. Terrified by this horrible disease, angry mobs would kill any individual thought to have helped spread it.

Colbert, Minister to Louis XIV, issued regulations for the whole of France in 1683 which gave a considerable amount of power to the Board of Health and quarantine station in Marseilles. Houses where individuals had contracted the plague were burned to the ground. In Milan, a writer who wiped his ink-stained fingers on the walls of houses he passed, was stripped, shaved, purged and then tortured. His right hand was cut off, he was stretched on the wheel, his bones were broken and his body was burned. Finally his ashes were thrown into the river and his belongings were all burnt. A servant girl in Germany who infected herself and her master with the plague by bringing infected property into their home in Königsberg died, but angry, frightened townsfolk ensured that she was exhumed, hanged and then burned at the foot of the gallows.

In the English village of Faversham, the local council appointed three wardens to examine people trying to enter the town and to exclude those who had come from well-known plague areas. A woman was paid to search for dead bodies, which were then buried in lime-filled pits. Infected clothing was burnt in huge fires which were never allowed to go out.

36

In 1667, Sir William Petty introduced a plan to reduce plagues in London which was based on the far-sighted economic argument for a medical service provided by the State. Petty suggested that the value to society of a healthy individual far exceeded the cost of providing a basic health service to the State and of organising a form of preventive medicine.

Petty was a well-known and respected renaissance man. Born in 1623, Petty was an English economist and statistician but he also studied medicine at Leyden, Paris and Oxford and worked as a Professor of Music, Professor of Anatomy and Member of Parliament. He argued that sanitary reform and health care could be cost-effective. His status didn't help much. His suggestions were largely ignored.

In the end, the plague died away not as a result of any human intervention but for reasons of its own. Epidemiologists are still puzzled by the way the disease seemed to disappear from Europe, making one last attack on Marseilles in 1720, when fifty thousand people were killed, and then disappearing until the end of the nineteenth century.

Some historians argue that the plague was transmitted by fleas which lived on the black rat and that it disappeared when the black rat was driven out of Europe by the brown rat, which has a different flea and does not live so close to human beings. Others claim that the black rat was still common in London after the end of the plague. They suggest that the plague was spread directly from man to man and that its demise was due to an acquired immunity which helped to protect the population.

We shall probably never know why the plague finally died away. But whatever the reason, it is unlikely to have had anything to do with medicine or the medical profession. (Nor, incidentally, is there much real support for the popular theory that the Great Fire of London cleansed that city.)

The disappearance of the plague was accompanied by other changes in the incidence of disorders that had previously been endemic in Europe. Leprosy which had at one time affected thousands throughout Europe, had more or less disappeared by the end of the sixteenth century, and syphilis, which had at first decimated the population in some parts of Europe, slowly began to fade in significance.

Other infectious disorders remained rife.

Influenza was common on both sides of the Atlantic, smallpox was seen everywhere, while dysentery and typhoid killed millions.

The death rate among mothers and infants remained high and half the newborn babies in seventeenth century England failed to survive. It was the high mortality rate among infants which kept life expectation figures low.

Much later, drug companies and doctors claimed that it was their work which pushed up life expectation figures. In truth, it was the infant mortality rate which kept average life expectation low. (If one person dies at or around birth and another individual lives to be 100, the average life span is 50 years. If both survive and live to the age of 75 the average life span is 75 years.)

In reality it wasn't until Dr John Snow removed the handle from the Broad Street pump that the medical profession made any progress in the control of infections.

Oliver Wendell Holmes (1809-1894)

In the early sixteenth century, Girolamo Fracastoro had suggested that infection might be caused by micro-organisms, and in the seventeenth century, Leeuwenhoek had seen these minute organisms under one of his microscopes. Sadly, however, the fact that unhygienic habits might be related to the spread of micro-organisms, and the consequent spread of disease, seems to have escaped observers until well into the nineteenth century.

One disease that had always been closely associated with hospitals was puerperal fever, a disorder which affects women after childbirth and which Hippocrates had recognised as being both fatal and contagious. The first doctor to recognise that puerperal fever might be prevented by keeping the maternity ward as clean as possible was a Manchester surgeon called Charles White who practised in the late eighteenth century. Unfortunately for several million women, White's observations and recommendations attracted little attention, and lying-in wards remained dirty, dangerous places until well into the nineteenth century.

In 1843, the American poet, novelist, anatomist and lecturer Oliver Wendell Holmes read to the Boston Society for Medical Improvement a paper *On the Contagiousness of Puerperal Fever,* in which he explained his theory that the disease can be carried from patient to patient by doctors themselves.

Holmes recommended that pregnant women in labour should not be attended by doctors who had been in contact with possible sources of infection. He specifically suggested that women having babies should not be attended by doctors who had come from conducting post-mortem examinations or dealing with cases of puerperal fever. He suggested that infection could be transmitted from one patient to another. Holmes also suggested that surgeons should consider changing their clothes and washing their hands in calcium chloride after leaving a patient with puerperal fever.

Despite the sense of his remarks, Holmes's controversial ideas annoyed a large part of the medical establishment, and his advice was ignored completely. There was violent opposition on the part of two powerful obstetricians working in Philadelphia (they were called Hodge and Meigs and like so many establishment figures, they are now remembered only for their pig headedness) but despite this, Holmes was brave enough to produce a monograph on the subject in 1855.

In a small book entitled *Puerperal Fever as a Private Pestilence* he repeated his views and pointed out that someone he described as 'Senderein' had lessened the mortality of puerperal fever by disinfecting his hands with chloride of lime and a nail-brush.

The Senderein to whom he referred was actually Ignaz Philipp Semmelweis.

Ignaz Semmelweis (1815-1865)

In 1846, a young physician called Ignaz Philipp Semmelweis, who was twenty-eight, became an assistant in one of the obstetric wards at the Allgemeines Krankenhaus in Vienna. The young Semmelweis noticed that the number of women dying in his ward was considerably higher than that in another obstetric ward at the hospital. Indeed, the difference was so noticeable that women frequently begged in tears not to be taken into Semmelweis's ward.

Deciding that the difference in the number of deaths had to be due to something other than the quality of his own clinical skills, Semmelweis looked for an explanation. He decided that the difference was that the ward with the better survival rate was looked after by the hospital's midwives, while in his own ward medical students assisted the obstetricians with deliveries.

Semmelweis then discovered that students came into the ward straight from the dissecting room and often performed intimate examinations with hands which only minutes before had been delving into corpses. The midwives, on the other hand, never went near the dissecting room and. on the contrary, had been taught that cleanliness was an important part of obstetric care.

Semmelweis's theory that the women were contracting puerperal fever from the students was strengthened when he attended a post mortem on another doctor in the hospital. This unfortunate man, a Dr Kolletschka, had died from a wound he had received in the dissecting room, and when his body was opened, Semmelweis noticed that the internal pathological signs were similar to those seen in women with puerperal fever.

Convinced that his theory about the spread of infection was correct, Semmelweis insisted that students and doctors coming from the dissecting room should wash their hands in a solution of calcium chloride before examining female patients. The precautions he introduced produced a dramatic drop in the number of deaths on his ward, from one in ten to approximately one in a hundred within two years.

Like Oliver Wendell Holmes, Semmelweis was viciously attacked by his colleagues at the hospital and by many other eminent obstetricians, who disagreed with his theory, despite its dramatic proof. Unable to cope with the opposition, Semmelweis left Vienna for Budapest, where he eventually became Professor of Obstetrics.

Unfortunately, the pressure brought about by the controversy proved too much for this mild and thoughtful man and he died in a mental hospital a few years later.

The history of medicine is full of men whose original work has been ignored or condemned by the establishment of the day.

Ignaz Semmelweis never knew but his courage and persistence eventually led directly to changes in medical practice which resulted in massive improvements in the quality of obstetric care throughout the world.

John Snow (1813-1858)

Dr John Snow was almost certainly the most influential of all British physicians and one of the most significant in world history. Snow made two huge contributions to medical practice.

First, he introduced anaesthesia into medical practice, and, in particular, for women in confinement. Second, by removing the handle from the Broad Street pump in Soho, he helped prevent the spread of cholera in London.

I have managed to obtain a complete copy of John Snow's personal casebooks which include, in amazing detail, his daily medical work from 17th July 1848 until March 5th 1858 (just under three months before his death at the age of 45) and they make extraordinary reading.

Anaesthesia was first used in Britain, on 19th December 1846, by a dentist called James Robinson, who practised in London and who should be remembered as one of the great heroes of medical and dental practice but who is, sadly, largely forgotten. (The man usually credited with being the first to discover and then promote anaesthesia was William Thomas Green Morton, also a dentist, who administered ether to a patient on 30th September 1846 and then removed a tooth without the patient suffering any pain. Historians point out that a surgeon called Crawford Williamson Long had apparently used ether as an anaesthetic four years earlier but didn't publish his findings until 1849. As many scientists have discovered to their cost, he who is first to publish will be the one to be remembered.)

Within days of hearing about this new development, Dr John Snow had tottered round to Robinson's home to find out more. The two men not only realised the importance of the discovery but also realised that if it were to be used effectively, the new speciality would need a scientific foundation.

Sadly, not all medical practitioners were as wise as Robinson and Snow and, in those early days, when anaesthetics were used in a very hit and miss sort of way, many of London's leading surgeons decided that anaesthesia was useless and dangerous. Robert Liston, who was the most famous surgeon operating in London, abandoned it and went back to operating on his patients while they were fully conscious. History does not record how his patients felt about this.

Snow, however, began to keep careful records of every patient he saw and to study the various methods by which anaesthetic 'vapours' could be administered. Pretty well single-handedly he turned anaesthesia into a science.

In 1848, Snow published a small textbook on the use of ether as an anaesthetic. His book is now regarded as a classic. During that same year Snow also started to use chloroform as an anaesthetic.

Inevitably, however, despite the evidence Snow produced, anaesthesia was slow to catch on. There was much opposition and, true to form, the medical establishment was slow to accept that putting patients to sleep during surgery might be a 'good idea'. (Again, no one bothered to ask patients what they thought about it.)

The level of opposition to anaesthetics can be judged from the fact that it wasn't until the 7th April 1853 that Dr Snow was invited to attend Queen Victoria during her confinement and to ease her pains with 53 minutes of chloroform. Afterwards, using a brand new pen nib, and in his best handwriting, Snow reported that the Queen 'appeared very cheerful and well, expressing herself much gratified with the effects of the chloroform'.

If the medical establishment had not been so slow to recommend anaesthesia, Queen Victoria would have been able to take advantage of Dr Snow's skills during the births of Princess Helena on 25th May 1848 and Prince Arthur on 1st May 1850.

Introducing anaesthesia into medical practice might have been enough for most practitioners but it was by no means enough for Dr Snow, who is also remembered as the most significant epidemiologist of his time and by some, of all time.

Between the years of 1846 and 1860, a cholera pandemic had killed people all over the world and there was still no agreement as to the cause, let alone agreement on a remedy. It was generally thought, however, that particles in the air were responsible for the spread of the disease.

It was in London during that epidemic that the relationship between cholera and water supplies was first proved.

Deciding that the only explanation for the way the disease seemed to spread was that it was carried in water supplies, Snow argued that the solution was to keep sewage away from drinking-water. He considered that, because the commonest symptoms of diarrhoea and vomiting, both involved the alimentary tract, the disease must be transmitted by something ingested rather than something carried in the air. He argued that an airborne contaminant would enter the lungs rather than the alimentary tract.

In 1849, when the second cholera outbreak hit London, Snow gave up his general practice in order to investigate his theory. At that time, piped water was not supplied to all houses in the area, and the people took their water from pumps and wells.

On 31st August 1854, a major outbreak of cholera occurred in Soho, London, and over three days 127 people who lived in or near to Broad Street died. During the next week, three quarters of the population had left the area. By the 10th September there had been 500 deaths. (As a matter of interest, many of the patients were taken to nearby Middlesex Hospital where Florence Nightingale had joined the hospital to help with the outbreak.)

A pump in Broad Street supplied the majority of local inhabitants, and Snow decided that the cholera epidemic in the area was linked directly to the use of the Broad Street pump.

A later investigation showed that the brick lining of a cesspool about three feet away from the well was cracked and decayed, and it seems likely that this was responsible for contaminating the previously drinkable water from the Broad Street pump. However, Snow also discovered that the local water company was taking its supplies from sewage polluted stretches of the river Thames and this was also a contributory factor. (Incidentally, none of the workers in the nearby Broad Street brewery contracted cholera because they were given a daily allowance of beer and did not, therefore, drink the water.)

The remarkable thing is that Snow had developed a simple epidemiological measure for controlling and preventing cholera some 30 years before the bacterium causing the disease had been identified.

Dr Snow persuaded the local parish authorities to disable the pump by removing the handle. The number of cholera deaths then fell.

To prevent the further spread of cholera, Snow recommended that the pump's handle be removed so that water could no longer be drawn.

The evidence was complete when Snow began to compare the incidence of cholera in areas of London supplied by different water companies. He found, for example, that customers of the Southwark and Vauxhall Water Company, which supplied water from the polluted lower reaches of the River Thames, were far more likely to get cholera than customers of the Lambeth Water Company, which took its water from a pure source.

Snow concluded that contaminated water was the source of the cholera and the reason for its spread. Moreover, he believed that a germ cell that had not yet been identified was the cause.

Inevitably, Snow's theory was furiously opposed by the medical establishment. London's leading medical officer at the time, Dr John Simon, described the germ theory which Snow espoused as 'peculiar' and the Board of Health in London dismissed Snow's theory completely and decided that the epidemic was due to miasma (particles in the air caused by decomposing matter). There can be little doubt that if the safety of the London population had been left in their hands the population of London would have been wiped out.

With the usual respect which local authorities show to heroes who are neither military nor political, no statue was erected to Snow and he was not given any honours. Indeed, with the callous disregard for history which has long characterised English councils, London County Council, ignored history and changed the name of this famous street to Broadwick Street in 1936. The only memorial to one of the most significant medical men in history is a public house which changed its name to the John Snow in 1955. This tribute is rather ironic since Snow was an ardent teetotaller for most of his life.

Epidemiology (the branch of medicine dealing with the incidence, distribution and control of disease) is, I believe, the most under-rated medical speciality. It is a tragedy that today it often seems to have been commandeered by mathematical modellers whose flights of fancy, derived from a superficial understanding of medical practice, frequently lead to grotesquely absurd and damaging predictions.

Michael Servetus (c1511-1553) and William Harvey (1578-1657)

Theories about the circulation of the blood had been proposed, argued and refuted by scientists and physicians of almost every era. Speculation had for many years been based on Galen's belief that the blood circulating in the arteries was different from the blood circulating in the veins, that both kinds of blood ebbed and flowed rather than circulated around the body and that blood permeated within the heart from the right side to the left.

Galen's claims misled medical scientists for many generations.

For some years before Harvey published his monograph *De Motu Cordis* in 1628, scientists had made educated guesses about the functions and actions of human blood. Theories were advanced in Italy by Colombo and Cesalpino, and in Spain by Michael Servetus.

Servetus wrote a book suggesting (accurately) that a separate pulmonary circulation existed within the body. For sharing this truth with the world, Servetus was burnt alive in 1553 by the Protestant leader John Calvin.

If Wikipedia had been around at the time, the editors would have doubtless called Servetus a conspiracy theorist and labelled him as discredited.

It wasn't until three quarters of a century later that anyone dared to take on the medical establishment with a theory about the workings of the heart.

An English physician and anatomist called William Harvey was the first person to produce experimental proof for his theory that since the heart was pumping blood along with every beat, it must be moving the blood somewhere.

It seems obvious to us now that the blood had to be moving around the body in a closed circulatory system, but that single, simple conclusion earned William Harvey immortality.

Harvey's original thinking and his ability to prove his ideas led to many changes in medical research and practical care. He explained his theory in his book *Exercitatio anatomica de motu cordis et sanguinis*, which was wisely dedicated to Charles I.

Harvey's theory that blood is pumped around the body in a continuous cycle led directly to the discovery of many other basic physiological facts. It also slowly led to the realisation that blood loss during operations could be fatal and that blood-letting, by leeching or cupping, was not always an entirely logical procedure. It also helped to refute the theory that weakness and blood loss could be remedied by drinking human blood – a belief which had survived until the fifteenth century, when Pope Innocent VIII had been given fresh blood from three healthy young boys to drink.

Jacques Cartier (1491-1557) and James Lind (1716-1794)

In 1535, Jacques Cartier had sailed from St. Malo in France with a total crew of 110 men, intending to explore the coast of Newfoundland, but within six weeks one hundred of his men had developed scurvy, a disease caused by the absence of Vitamin C from the diet. In the early stages the symptoms are simple enough – the patient usually notices that his gums bleed rather easily. Later on, however, the disorder begins to affect the whole body, resulting in considerable pain before death intervenes.

Luckily for his men and his expedition, Cartier discovered from a native that the complaint could be cured by drinking the juice from the fruit of local trees. His crew recovered within days.

Wise sea captains quickly followed Cartier's example and, to maintain a healthy crew, ensured that each man was provided with a regular supply of either orange or lemon juice. In a book called *The Surgeon's Mate,* published in 1636, John Woodall recommended that these juices be used to prevent the development of scurvy. He didn't know why the fruit juices worked – but he knew that they did.

Nevertheless, the establishment refused to accept this simple truth and remarkably and inexplicably, captains stopped providing their crews with citrus fruits. As a result, scurvy began once again to decimate crews on long voyages. When Anson's fleet circumnavigated the globe between 1740 and 1744, he lost three quarters of his men to scurvy.

It was not until 1747 that the idea of preventing scurvy by giving sailors lemon or orange juice to drink was reintroduced.

The man who suggested it was James Lind, an Edinburgh graduate, who performed the·first proper clinic trial in his successful attempt to prove that, by using one or other of these fruits, scurvy could be prevented. Lind published the results from his study in 1753 and described how he had given some sailors vinegar, some cider, some oranges and some lemons. Only those sailors who had been given fruit avoided scurvy.

Despite this evidence, the Admiralty still refused to act and in the Seven Years' War, from 1756 to 1763, approximately half of the 185,000 sailors involved died of scurvy,

Lind's work did enable a young Lieutenant Cook (later to be promoted) to sail around the world between 1769 and 1771 without a single case of scurvy but surprisingly, the Admiralty still took no notice of Lind's research and in 1779 the Channel Fleet had 2,400 cases of scurvy after a ten week cruise.

However, Sir Gilbert Blane cured an outbreak on twenty eight ships in 1782 by using fruit and eventually succeeded in convincing the Admiralty chiefs that the proposal was worth following.

In 1795, a year after Lind's death, lemon juice became a compulsory part of every sailor's diet. To make sure that the sailors took their lemon, it was added to their grog ration. When, in later years, limes were used instead of lemons, the Americans gave British sailors the nickname 'limey' to commemorate the fact.

It was perhaps just as well that the Admiralty acted when it did. It is unlikely that even Nelson's tactical skills could have made up for a navy decimated by scurvy, and the wars with Napoleon which were to follow might have had a rather different outcome.

Philippe Pinel (1745-1826)

At the beginning of the eighteenth century Daniel Defoe, best remembered for his account of the exploits of Robinson Crusoe, had written a bitter complaint about the number of private mad-houses where, for a decent fee, patients could be hidden away from the world.

'Is it not enough to make anyone mad,' he asked 'to be suddenly clap'd up, stripp'd, whipp'd, ill fed and worse us'd? To have no reason assigned for such treatment, no crime alleged or accusers to confront? And what is worse, no soul to appeal to but merciless creatures who answer but in laughter, surliness, contradiction and too often stripes?'

But no one in Europe took much notice of Defoe, and medical practitioners continued to treat mentally ill patients in the belief that physical punishments would cure their troubles.

At London's Bethlem Royal Hospital, known better as Bedlam, half-naked patients were kept chained in irons, were allowed only straw bedding and were cruelly mistreated. Physicians bled their patients at the end of May or the beginning of June each year, and after being bled, each patient would be made to vomit once a week before being purged. For the more troublesome patients there was a tranquillising wheel on which individuals could be strapped and spun round until they lost consciousness. Until 1770, visitors could pay a penny to see the 'fun' at Bedlam.

To put this in perspective, it should be remembered that general hospitals were not much better than hospitals catering for the mentally ill. In 1788, Jacobus-René Tenon published a report describing the hospitals of Paris which must have shocked even the most complacent city officials. He described how the Hotel Dieu contained 1,220 beds, in each of which between four and six patients were crammed. Patients in many parts of the hospital lay about on dirty straw, and no attempt was made to keep infectious patients away from those suffering from non-infectious diseases. The stench in the hospital was said to be so foul that people entering it would

51

often do so only when holding a vinegar-soaked sponge to their noses. Patients who had surgical operations invariably died, and relatively few patients ever walked out of the hospital. Most healthy pregnant women confined in the Hotel Dieu died in childbirth. The same things were true of almost all other hospitals throughout Europe. When Tsar Paul came to power in Russia in 1796, he was so horrified at the state of the hospital in Moscow that he ordered it to be rebuilt. In Frankfurt physicians considered working in hospital equivalent to a sentence of death. Another reforming writer of the eighteenth century, John Howard, toured European hospitals and prisons at about the same time as Tenon made his report, and his studies were equally startling. It was the same story almost everywhere: dirty straw as bedding, no fresh air, no sunlight, no bandages and a milk and water diet supplemented with weak soup.

It was only when Florence Nightingale returned from the Crimea as a hero that general hospitals changed. Before Miss Nightingale took a small group of nurses to the Crimea, the death rate among the wounded at Scutari had been forty-two per cent. After her arrival, it fell to two per cent. There could have been no better proof of the efficacy of the 'Nightingale' methods. When she returned from the Crimea, Florence Nightingale was a national heroine. Her uncompromising attitude towards the reactionary military authorities on behalf of the sick and wounded British soldiers had proved so popular that the staggering sum of £50,000 was raised on her behalf to found a school for nurses at St. Thomas's Hospital in London. The nurses who qualified there spread 'the Gospel according to Florence' to other major British hospitals, and within a few years every major hospital had its own training school. In a comparatively short time, the nursing profession was established as a respectable, worthwhile part of the medical profession. (There is more about Florence Nightingale, and other medical heroes, in my book *The Story of Medicine*.)

But if the standard of care in ordinary hospitals was low, that in mental hospitals and psychiatric institutions was almost beyond description or comprehension. At the Blockley Hospital in Philadelphia a report published in 1793 showed that, since it was almost impossible to hire nurses, insane, female patients were looked after by just three male keepers, who exhibited their patients as a sort of side-show, opening the wards to the public and allowing visitors to poke fun at the more obviously insane patients. There was no heating in the hospital because the authorities had decided that insane patients were unlikely to suffer from extremes of temperature. Dr Benjamin Rush, thought to have been one of the most enlightened medical practitioners in America, is reported to have kept disturbed patients awake and standing for twenty-four hours at a time.

John Wesley, the founder of the Wesleyan Church, suggested that a useful treatment for lunacy might include rubbing the patient's head several times a day with vinegar in which ground ivy leaves had been infused. More seriously ill patients, described by him as suffering from raving madness, would receive more dramatic remedies, and he pointed out that, since all madmen were cowards, binding them sometimes did as much good as beating. Wesley, who seems to have considered himself a benefactor of the mentally ill, also suggested pouring water onto their heads and giving them a diet of nothing but apples for a month. Between these treatments, mental patients would usually be confined to over-crowded quarters where urine-soaked and excrement-laden straw would serve as bedding. Wesley, incidentally, was one of the first men to use electricity in the attempted treatment of mental illness.

One of the most powerful indictments of the ways in which the mentally ill were cared for was made by Dr Philippe Pinel, a physician to Bicêtre and Salpêtrière prisons in Paris, where many lunatics were housed.

Pinel decided to offer to free a number of prisoners from their chains if they promised to behave like gentlemen. To the surprise of the less imaginative officials, the prisoners were not violent or disorderly when their chains were removed.

Like Hippocrates many years before, Pinel argued that the mentally ill are sick and not responsible for their condition. Pinel amplified this simple theory in a textbook written in 1801, which was effectively the first treatise on psychiatry. He created the first classification of mental illness and described how mental illnesses can be temporary or permanent and either relapsing or persistent. He also argued that domestic crises, unhappy love affairs and similar stresses can all produce types of mental illness.

Unfortunately, not everyone agreed with Pinel, and the humane theories he had expressed were not widely accepted for many years. Pinel's humanitarian approach to mental illness was criticised by the nurses in the hospitals where he worked, and he was also criticised for suggesting that a patient's environmental and social problems might be responsible for their mental illness. Senior members of the medical profession preferred to believe that mental health issues were a result of brain lesions.

And so, sadly, at the beginning of the nineteenth century, mental hospitals were still quite unsuitable for the care of people needing medical attention and it wasn't until the middle of the 19th century, long after Pinel's death, that there was any real, widespread improvement in the care of the mentally ill.

Franz Mesmer (1734-1815)

Of the many so-called quacks who made major contributions to medical science, the one who probably stands above the rest was Franz Mesmer.

Mesmer graduated in Vienna in 1766 and aroused the sort of controversy that had first surrounded Paracelsus two centuries earlier. Mesmer began his academic career by studying the power and influence of the universe on human beings, and his first theory was that some unseen power from the planets influenced human behaviour in just the same way as the moon influences the sea. At first, Mesmer believed that the power was transmitted through ordinary magnets, since his experiments suggested that by moving a magnet he could control the flow of fluid from a patient being bled, but gradually he began to realise that the magnet was not really necessary and that the same effect could be obtained with nothing more mysterious than his own hands. 'Hypnosis', in its various forms (the word 'hypnosis' had not then been invented), had been the subject of study and experimentation since the days of ancient Egypt and Athanasius Kircher, a seventeenth century microscopist, had done some significant work on the subject, but Mesmer was the first man to seek to use the influence of the mind over the body.

Mesmer claimed that the explanation for this new power source was something called 'animal magnetism', a powerful basic force derived from the planets or from some other unknown body in space, which could be utilised by human hands and controlled in such a way as to have an effect on individual patients.

His theories might have been debatable but there was no doubt that Mesmer was enormously successful and the Austrian medical establishment quickly started a campaign to discredit him. When he cured a young blind girl, they accused him of being a cheat and a charlatan.

Thrown out of Vienna, Mesmer moved to Paris, where he soon established an even more lucrative private practice. Undoubtedly quite a showman, Mesmer would dress up for his séances and influence his patients with music, staring eyes and a wand. For a while he continued to use magnets as part of his consulting room technique, although he realised and openly admitted that they were not necessary. His success with patients suffering from disorders which we would now describe as 'psychosomatic' or 'stress induced' was tremendous.

Inevitably, Mesmer's success in Paris once again aroused considerable controversy, and many members of the medical establishment, inspired no doubt more by jealousy than other motives, set up a special commission to investigate his claims. The commissioners, who included Benjamin Franklin, the chemist Lavoisier and a Dr Guillotin, who invented the instrument which bears his name, decided that there was no justification for any such force as animal magnetism and instead claimed that Mesmer's cures were produced by the patient's imagination. It didn't seem to occur to them that *how* Mesmer's patients were cured didn't matter as much as the fact that they were.

Whether or not the commission's findings would have affected his practice we have no way of knowing, for Mesmer was not to be in Paris for much longer. The King, Louis XVI, and his court had been enthusiastic supporters of Mesmerism, and when the French Revolution became a reality, Mesmer left France.

Although he died in obscurity in Switzerland in 1815, Mesmer's influence on medical care and, in particular, on the treatment of the mentally ill remains important. His ability to control, influence and cure the mentally ill helped lead to reforms in practical psychiatry, and such men as Sigmund Freud owed a great deal to his work.

Although the medical establishment considered him to be a quack and a showman, Franz Mesmer was probably one of the most influential and important figures in the history of eighteenth century medicine.

Margaret Sanger (1883-1966) and Marie Stopes (1880-1958)

The greatest impact in the field of birth control was made by two women.

In America, the fight to provide contraceptive advice was led by Margaret Sanger.

In Europe one of the most important campaigners was Marie Stopes.

These two women, both determined feminists, were together responsible for the introduction and organisation of birth control clinics and for the dissemination of advice and equipment.

Margaret Sanger, herself the sixth of eleven children, began her career as a nurse in New York City, where she saw at first hand the close links between poverty, large families and disease. There were at that time, in America, laws forbidding the promotion of any information about contraception, and so when, in 1914, Mrs Sanger published a magazine and a pamphlet including details about contraception, she was arrested. That case was dismissed, but in 1916, when she opened the first birth-control clinic, she was charged with 'maintaining a public nuisance' and sent to the workhouse for thirty days. (Mrs Sanger invented the phrase birth-control'.) The publicity aroused by the case and the furore that followed other similar battles eventually led to a relaxation of the law.

Marie Stopes, born three years earlier than Margaret Sanger, in 1880, qualified as a botanist in Munich and taught her subject at Manchester University, until the failure of her marriage led her to a study of the problems of matrimony. Her research in this area led her to believe that birth control could help to save some marriages, and in 1921 she founded Britain's first birth-control clinic.

The opposition which Sanger and Stopes faced came mainly from the Church, and in particular from the Roman Catholic Church, which considered contraception of any kind to be a sin.

Technically, Margaret Sanger and Marie Stopes had only the simplest forms of contraceptives to offer; intra-uterine devices were available only to a very small number of women, oral contraceptives did not come onto the market until the 1950s, and sterilisation did not become popular until surgical techniques had made it a simple and relatively painless operation.

But, despite considerable opposition, social and political attitudes towards birth control were formed in those early years of the twentieth century when the establishment was confronted by two very determined women: one in America and one in Europe.

Alexander Fleming (1881-1955)

Alexander Fleming's discovery of penicillin in 1928 was as much the result of good fortune as of careful planning. Serendipity has always played a larger part in medical progress than most doctors like to admit but in Fleming's case indifference and a lack of imagination were responsible for the fact that his discovery, vitally important as it was, lay unused for many years.

According to the now well-established legend, Fleming had been working in his laboratory at St. Mary's Hospital in London on a study of the staphylococcus bacteria when he noticed that a culture dish containing the bacteria appeared to have been contaminated and the contaminant had in some way stopped the growth of the bacteria.

In retrospect it seems likely that someone had left a laboratory window open through which spores of a common fungus had blown. (Historians have argued about this, and while some agree with the window theory, others say that the spores entered through a door, while a third group claim that the spores reached the culture dish through a ventilation shaft. I find it difficult to get excited about where the contaminant came from.)

Contamination is a common problem in laboratories, and normally such cultures are simply thrown away.

Fleming, however, like Röntgen (who accidentally discovered X-rays) and so many others, was too good a scientist just to toss away the contents of the dish and forget about the incident. He made careful notes on the culture, and the following year published a paper in the *British Journal of Experimental Pathology* describing the way in which the growing spores (which he had identified as being those of penicillium notarum) had contaminated the culture dish and prevented the growth of the bacteria. Tests showed that the penicillin mould was safe for human use, and Fleming realised that one day it would prove useful as a drug, but he found that it was too unstable to be manufactured in any quantity.

And that was that. None of the experts within the medical establishment spotted the significance of the discovery, and

Fleming's work on penicillin was to lie untouched for a decade. During that period, however, research for effective anti-infective agents made progress in Germany. In 1932, Gerhard Domagk, a director at the Bayer Laboratory for Experimental Pathology and Bacteriology in Wuppertal-Elberfeld, who had been experimenting on new dyes and drugs, decided to investigate a new wool dye, prontosil red, to evaluate its use as a drug.

The story goes that Domagk's daughter, Hildegarde, had pricked her finger with a knitting needle and had developed blood poisoning at just about the time that the therapeutic effect of prontosil was discovered, and that in an attempt to save her, Domagk decided to try the new drug. The drug worked, and realising the commercial value of a synthetic product which could be used to combat infection, many of the world's major drug companies began work in attempts to develop similar products. (One of the products which resulted from this international search was M & B 693, an anti-bacterial developed by a company called May & Baker which was used to treat a patient called Winston Churchill when he developed pneumonia during the Second World War.)

The success of prontosil encouraged other scientists to dig out Fleming's discovery and begin work on penicillin.

The next vital step took place in Oxford, where a team of scientists led by Professor Howard Florey and Dr Ernst Chain solved the problem of how to manufacture penicillin in a stable form. Their research coincided with the outbreak of the Second World War, and when it was realised that the new drug would be an important asset to any army, many scientists and drug companies on both sides of the Atlantic began to study ways of manufacturing penicillin in large quantities. By the end of the war, thanks to the combined efforts of British and American manufacturers, penicillin was being produced with comparative ease. (Undoubtedly the drug's military significance resulted in its large-scale production being achieved at an earlier date than would otherwise have been the case.)

During the years following Ehrlich's first discovery, many drugs were produced, and in recent years the production of new compounds has reached almost epidemic proportions.

In the 1930s, before antibiotics were widely available, the number of people dying from pneumonia in the United States sometimes exceeded fifty per cent of those who had contracted the infection.

After the introduction of antibiotics, the death rate fell to about one in twenty. Similar improvements were noticed with other infectious disorders. Once general practitioners were able to provide prescriptions for antibiotics, the number of people needing prolonged bed rest or nursing care for the duration of an infective illness also fell.

Antibiotic drugs were the most important weapons to be added to the doctor's armoury in the twentieth century, but the medical establishment can take very little credit for them.

Dean Ornish (1953-)

An American physician called Dr Dean Ornish has done astonishing work in the treatment of patients with heart disease and cancer.

First, Ornish showed that it is actually possible to treat patients with existing heart disease by encouraging them to make significant changes in the way they live. Dr Ornish was the first clinician to provide documented proof that heart disease can be halted or even reversed simply by a change in life-style. After one year, the majority (82%) of the patients who made the comprehensive lifestyle changes recommended by Dr Ornish showed some measurable reversal of their coronary artery blockages.

Dr Ornish and his colleagues showed that by persuading patients to follow some simple basic rules – which include taking half an hour's moderate exercise every day, spending at least an hour a day practising relaxation and stress management techniques and following a low fat vegetarian diet, they could frequently help get rid of coronary artery blockages and heart pain. Their work was, of course, not popular with heart surgeons or drug companies, of course. Sadly, I'm afraid that the potential for making money out of this sort of 'commonsense' regime is far too slight to please the medical establishment.

If your doctor hasn't heard of the non- surgical, non-drug treatment of heart disease, it is probably because he or she obtains all his or her post-graduate medical information from drug company sponsored lectures and publications.

Dr Ornish isn't the only doctor to have produced important work in this area. In a review entitled, *The Natural Cure of Coronary Heart Disease* (published in the journal *'Nutrition and Health'* in 2003) Dr Allan Withnell concluded that the medical literature: 'strongly suggests that lifestyle and particularly diet are the cause and the cure of coronary heart disease. The proof will lie in persuading the cardiac patient to change his lifestyle to the extent recommended and observing the result.' Dr Withnell has put emphasis on the words 'to the extent recommended' and his point is important. It's no good just cutting down from two burgers a day to one.

Dr Ornish, Director of the Preventive Medicine Research Unit in Sausalito California and Clinical Professor of Medicine at the University of California, San Francisco, has also shown that prostate cancer be treated with a simple regime which consists of moderate exercise, a vegan diet and stress relaxation techniques. Writing in the *Journal of Urology* in 2005, Dr Ornish showed that patients who followed this regime rigorously, saw their prostate antigen scores drop. Blood serum taken from patients on this programme inhibited cancer cells eight times as much as serum from other patients. There seems no doubt that green vegetables and lycopene provide protection against cancer-promoting chemicals.

A total of 93 men who had proven prostate cancer and who had (for their own reasons) chosen not to undergo conventional treatment were divided into two groups. One group were asked not to make any changes in their lifestyle or diet. The other group were asked to make comprehensive changes.

The men in the second group were placed on a vegan diet which consisted primarily of fruits, vegetables, whole grains and legumes supplemented with soy, vitamins and minerals. They took part in modern aerobic exercise, yoga or meditation and were placed in a weekly support group. None of these men had any conventional treatment such as surgery, radiation or chemotherapy.

Dr Ornish's work showed clearly that men with early stage prostate cancer (cancer which had not spread throughout their bodies) who made intensive changes in their lifestyle and diet were able to stop or reverse the progression of their disease. The study showed that 453 genes linked to cancer were 'turned off' and 48 protective genes were 'turned on' for the patients who followed the programme of exercise, diet and stress management. There is growing and convincing evidence that cutting down on saturated fat and increasing the consumption of vegetables, fruit and fibre can help prevent prostate cancer from developing or recurring. Since breast cancer is also often dependent upon hormone levels it seems likely that breast cancer must be similarly responsive to diet.

Despite the evidence, Dr Ornish's work (particularly his dietary programme) has been criticised, and doctors and hospitals continue to treat heart disease with drugs and surgery and to treat prostate cancer with drugs, radiotherapy or surgery or a combination of all three. In the United States, however, the Ornish programme has been authorised as a cardiac rehabilitation program by Medicare.

Professor T.Colin Campbell (1934-)

There is a considerable amount of evidence showing that patients who have cancer can at best cure themselves or at worst dramatically improve their odds of surviving if they stop eating animal proteins. In a book called *The China Study*, written by Professor T.Colin Campbell in 2005, the author argues that the main protein found in dairy products, a substance called casein, could be regarded as a Category 1 carcinogen and is the most significant carcinogen we consume.

The importance of diet has without a doubt been suppressed by people driven by a toxic mixture of self-interest, prejudice, laziness and greed. It is sad that many oncologists still fail to understand the importance of avoiding dairy produce.

The Memorial Sloan Kettering Cancer Centre publishes a 'Lifestyle and Breast Cancer Risk' list which points out that diet and lifestyle may play a role both in the development of breast cancer and its recurrence. They suggest that the key to avoiding both of these eventualities is achieving and maintaining a healthy body weight, eating a balanced, mostly plant based diet, exercising regularly, getting enough sleep and, pretty obviously, not smoking or drinking too much alcohol.

Sadly, none of this advice is offered by hospitals and doctors in the UK where surgery, chemotherapy and radiotherapy are still the preferred options.

Astonishingly, the official advice from the NHS is that all adults should consume lots of cow's milk because it is rich in calcium. This advice is offered despite the fact that researchers who studied 53,000 women over eight years, found that women who drank two cups of milk a day had an 80% increase in their risk of breast cancer. Even a third of a cup of milk a day increases the risk of cancer by 30%.

The truth, I fear, is that the Government dare not upset the powerful farming lobby and through carelessness, indifference or ignorance the medical establishment prefers to stick with its own self-serving options.

Afterword

The world of medicine today is just as hidebound and unwilling to accept significant discoveries as it has ever been. So-called experts, sitting comfortably within the medical establishment but paid by drug companies or lobby groups to promote commercial interests are regarded as the ultimate arbiters of what should or should not be done.

One common result is patients are widely mis-treated by being given drugs and vaccines which are known to cause serious health problems. There can be no doubt that millions of patients are regularly made worse by the treatment they receive.

Most worrying of all, perhaps, is the fact that many new products introduced by the pharmaceutical industry are never adequately tested for safety or efficacy. There is evidence, indeed, that products which are shown to cause serious health problems are frequently sold and widely promoted with the evidence of their harm being suppressed. Only when the evidence of malpractice becomes widespread are the products reluctantly withdrawn.

Appendix 1: Biography of the Author

Vernon Coleman was an angry young man for as long as it was decently possible. He then turned into an angry middle-aged man. And now, with no effort whatsoever, he has matured into being an angry old man. He is, he confesses, just as angry as he ever was. Indeed, he may be even angrier because, he says, the more he learns about life the more things he finds to be angry about.

Cruelty, prejudice and injustice are the three things most likely to arouse his well-developed sense of ire but he admits that, at a pinch, inefficiency, incompetence and greed will do almost as well.

The author has an innate dislike of taking orders, a pathological contempt for pomposity, hypocrisy and the sort of unthinking political correctness which attracts support from *Guardian* reading pseudo-intellectuals. He also has a passionate loathing for those in authority who do not understand that unless their authority is tempered with compassion and a sense of responsibility, the end result must always be an extremely unpleasant brand of totalitarianism.

Vernon Coleman qualified as a doctor in 1970 and has worked both in hospitals and as a principal in general practice. He has organised many campaigns concerning iatrogenesis, drug addiction and the abuse of animals and has given evidence to committees at the House of Commons and the House of Lords. Dr Coleman's campaigns have often proved successful. For example, after a 15 year campaign (which started in 1973) he eventually persuaded the British Government to introduce stricter controls governing the prescribing of benzodiazepine tranquillisers. 'Dr Vernon Coleman's articles, to which I refer with approval, raised concern about these important matters,' said the Parliamentary Secretary for Health in the House of Commons in 1988.

Coleman has worked as a columnist for numerous national newspapers including *The Sun, The Daily Star, The Sunday Express, The Sunday Correspondent* and *The People*. He once wrote three columns at the same time for national papers (he wrote them under three different names). At the same time he was also writing weekly columns for the *Evening Times* in Glasgow and for the *Sunday Scot*.

His syndicated columns have appeared in over 50 regional newspapers. His columns and articles have appeared in newspapers and magazines around the world. In the UK he has contributed articles and stories to hundreds of other publications including *The Sunday Times, Observer, Guardian, Daily Telegraph, Sunday Telegraph, Daily Express, Daily Mail, Mail on Sunday, Daily Mirror, Sunday Mirror, Punch, Woman, Woman's Own, The Lady, Spectator* and *British Medical Journal*. He was the founding editor of the *British Clinical Journal*.

For many years he wrote a monthly newsletter. He has lectured doctors and nurses on a variety of medical matters. Tens of millions have consulted his telephone advice lines, watched his videos and visited his websites.

He has presented numerous programmes on television and radio and was the original breakfast television doctor. He was television's first agony uncle (on BBC1's *The Afternoon Show*) and presented three TV series based on his bestselling book *Bodypower*. In the now long-gone days when producers and editors were less wary of annoying the establishment he was a regular broadcaster on many radio and television programmes.

In the 1980s he wrote the algorithms for the first computerised health programmes – which sold around the world (or, at least, in 26 countries) to those far-sighted individuals who had bought the world's first home computers.

His books have been published in the UK *by Arrow, Pan, Penguin, Corgi, Mandarin, Star, Piatkus, RKP, Thames and Hudson, Sidgwick and Jackson, Macmillan* and many other leading publishing houses and translated into 25 languages. English language versions sell in the USA, Australia, Canada and South Africa. Several of his books have appeared on both the *Sunday Times* and *Bookseller* bestseller lists. His books have sold over two million copies in the UK, been translated into 25 languages and now sell in over 50 countries. His bestselling non-fiction book *Bodypower* was voted one of the 100 most popular books of the 1980s/90s and was turned into two television series in the UK. His novel *Mrs Caldicot's Cabbage War* has been filmed and is, like many of his other novels, available in an audio version.

Coleman has written numerous books and articles under a vast variety of pennames (some of which he has now forgotten). When he feels tired (which happens with increasing frequency) his wife reminds him of all this and he sometimes feels better for a little while. Vernon

Coleman's work has also been included in many anthologies including the *Penguin Book of 21st Century Protest*. He has contributed to various encyclopaedias.

Vernon Coleman has worked for the Open University in the UK and was an honorary Professor of Holistic Medical Sciences at the Open International University based in Sri Lanka. He has received lots of rather jolly awards from people he likes and respects. He is, for example, a Knight Commander of The Ecumenical Royal Medical Humanitarian Order of Saint John of Jerusalem, a Knight Commander of the Knights of Malta and a member of the Ancient Royal Order of Physicians dedicated to His Majesty King Buddhadasa. In 2000, he was awarded the Yellow Emperor's Certificate of Excellence as Physician of the Millennium by the Medical Alternativa Institute.

He has never had a proper job (in the sense of working for someone else in regular, paid employment, with a cheque or pay packet at the end of the week or month) but he has had freelance and temporary employment in many forms. He has, for example, had employment as: postman, fish delivery van driver, production line worker, chemical laboratory assistant, author, publisher, draughtsman, meals on wheels driver, feature writer, drama critic, magician's assistant, book reviewer, columnist, surgeon, police surgeon, industrial medical officer, social worker, nightclub operator, property developer, magazine editor, general practitioner, private doctor, television presenter, radio presenter, agony aunt, university lecturer, casualty doctor and care home assistant.

In March 2020, and for the following two years, Coleman shared facts and inconvenient truths about global health events. As a result, his career and reputation were deliberately and systemically destroyed. He was banned from all mainstream media and the press, TV and radio published lies and libels about him. Editors he had known for years refused to speak to him.

Most damagingly he was lied about on Wikipedia, and several Wikipedia pages about his books and book series were removed. Google repeated the lies promoted on Wikipedia. Overnight, all his achievements were removed from Wikipedia. At least one of the editors named as responsible for altering his Wikipedia pages is, according to Larry Sanger (Wikipedia's co-founder) suspected of having links to the CIA.

Coleman was banned from Facebook, Twitter and Linkedin and all his videos were removed from YouTube (he had acquired over 200,000 subscribers in record time). His books were banned by internet publishers. All his books were banned in China (where they were bestsellers) and Germany (where they were bestsellers). He was expelled from the Royal Society of Arts (one of the reasons being that he had been attacked on a one sided, prejudiced BBC's Panorama programme on which he was attacked for telling the truth but not invited into the studio to defend himself.)

Fake channels in his name appeared on social media (e.g. Telegram – which failed to remove the fakes, and each month there are around 3,000 attempts to hack into/destroy each of his personal websites. The video platform BrandNewTube was told to stop him making videos or the platform would be closed down. Scores of self-appointed Factcheckers around the world lied about him and accused him of spreading misinformation without ever finding any factual errors in over 300 videos and around 1,000 articles which he had written about the 2020 frauds.

Today, he writes, reads and collects books and has a larger library than most towns. He has never been much of an athlete, though he once won a certificate for swimming a width of the public baths in Walsall and once swam a mile for charity. He finished after everyone else had gone home and had switched off the lights.

Vernon Coleman has co-written five books with his wife, Donna Antoinette Coleman who is a talented oil painter whose work has been exhibited. She is the author of *My Quirky Cotswold Garden*.

Vernon and Antoinette Coleman have been happily married for more than 20 years and they live in the delightful if isolated village of Bilbury in Devon where he and his wife have designed for themselves a unique world to sustain and nourish them in these dark and difficult times.

Vernon would like it to be known that he is devoted to Donna Antoinette who is the kindest, sweetest, most sensitive woman a man could hope to meet. He can ride a bicycle and swim, though not at the same time.

Appendix 2: References
Reference Articles referring to Vernon Coleman

Ref 1
'Volunteer for Kirkby' – *The Guardian,* 14.5.1965
(Article re VC's work in Kirkby, Liverpool as a Community Service
Volunteer in 1964-5)
Ref 2
'Bumbledom forced me to leave the NHS' – *Pulse*, 28.11.1981
(Vernon Coleman resigns as a GP after refusing to disclose
confidential information on sick note forms)
Ref 3
'I'm Addicted To The Star' – *The Star*, *10.3.1988*
Ref 4
'Medicine Becomes Computerised: Plug In Your Doctor.' – *The
Times*, 29.3.1983
Ref 5
'Computer aided decision making in medicine' – *British Medical
Journal*, 8.9.1984 and 27.10.1984
Ref 6
'Conscientious Objectors' – *Financial Times magazine,* 9.8.2003

Major interviews with Vernon Coleman include:
'Doctor with the Common Touch.' – *Birmingham Post*, 9.10.1984
'Sacred Cows Beware: Vernon Coleman publishing again.' – *The
Scotsman*, 6.12.1984
'Our Doctor Coleman Is Mustard' – *The Sun,* 29.6.1988
'Reading the mind between the lines.' – *BMA News Review,*
November 1991
Doctors' Firsts – *BMA News Review,* 21.2.1996
'The big league of self publishing.' – *Daily Telegraph,* 17.8.1996
'Doctoring the books' – *Independent,* 16.3.1999
'Sick Practices' – *Ode Magazine,* July/August 2003
'You have been warned, Mr Blair.' – *Spectator,* 6.3.2004 and
20.3.2004

'Food for thought with a real live Maverick.' – *Western Daily Press*, 5.9.2006

'The doctor will see you now' – *Independent*, 14.5.2008

There is a more comprehensive list of reference articles on www.vernoncoleman.com

Final Note from the Author

If you found this book informative I would be very grateful if you would put a suitable review online. It helps more than you can imagine. If you disliked the book, or disapproved of it in any way, please forget you read it.

Vernon Coleman

Printed in Great Britain
by Amazon

25459418R00050